CW01501959

DEMENTIA
CARE COMPANION

DEMENTIA
CARE COMPANION

THE **COMPLETE HANDBOOK** OF
PRACTICAL CARE
FROM **EARLY** TO **LATE** STAGE

MEHDI SAMADANI

COGNITIVIX PRESS
2022

Published by Cognitivix Press, San Jose, California.
www.cognitivixpress.com

Cognitivix Press and Cognitivix are trademarks or registered trademarks of Cognitivix Inc. All other trademarks are the property of their respective owners.

Cover Illustration: Elaheh Azarnoosh
Interior Illustrations: Richard Kear

Library of Congress Control Number: 2022943729
ISBN 979-8-9866677-0-6

To my wife
Whose battle with dementia brought
Unexpected moments of joy and togetherness,
And love and loss,
Every day

And

To caregivers around the world
Keepers of the light in silent sacrifice,
For weary loved ones to find their way home

You Will Make Mistakes

On this journey, no two days are the same. No two patients are the same, and no two problems are the same. You learn as you go, and sometimes, you learn too late. Learn to forgive yourself. Forgive early, and forgive often. Accept life as it comes. Plan ahead. Stay vigilant. Eliminate the risks that can be eliminated, and manage the ones that cannot. Do the best that you can, with what you have, given your individual circumstances. And then, accept that it will have to be enough.

CONTENTS

2 | FIRST STEPS

3 | PLANNING FOR EFFECTIVE CARE

4 | GETTING HELP 63

5 | DEMENTIA-FRIENDLY HOME 81

10 | COMMUNICATION

19 | MOBILITY AND BALANCE 307

LIST OF FIGURES

Our Story

Dementia doesn't aim for the patient alone;
It has its sights on the caregiver, too.

Our third appointment was on a hot July afternoon. We had seen our neurologist twice already, and had been to a number of tests and exams. An MRI of my wife's brain had shown atrophy in the frontal and temporal regions, and a subsequent PET scan was supposed to show the extent of activity or inactivity in those areas. Today, our neurologist would have the results for us.

Over the previous six months, my wife's condition had deteriorated. She'd be happy one moment, then crying the next. She'd stand in front of the bathroom mirror rehashing grievances and spiraling into despair until we'd intervene. Sometimes she'd be indifferent to people and events around her, and at other times she'd be her old loving, empathetic self again. When returning from our daily walks, she sometimes wouldn't recognize our home and would refuse to go inside. One time she couldn't find her car in the parking lot of the grocery store and believed it had been stolen. She wasn't sure of her memory anymore and asked for detailed directions to and from familiar places. She had forgotten how to use the TV and needed help turning it on...

We lived in San Jose, California. I had taken early retirement and was spending more and more time either handholding my wife, looking for answers in books and online, or pouring over long emails to and from our children debating and dissecting their mother's condition. We all knew we were facing a serious problem. We just didn't grasp the depth of what was yet to come.

At our appointment, the look on the doctor's face said it all. The diagnosis had been conclusive: my wife had frontotemporal dementia. He didn't go into much detail in front of her. Instead, he handed me a letter in which he had spelled it out: ... *progressive brain disorder... similar to Alzheimer's disease... loss of brain cells... two to ten years... no cure.* Privately, he told me that there was nothing more he could do for us. Other than medication to help manage some of the symptoms, there was no treatment available. I asked if there was anything else I should do. His answer surprised me.

"Take care of yourself," he said.

"Take care of *myself?*"

"Yes!"

He said that I was at risk. Someone would have to keep an eye on me and sound the alarm at the first warning signs of depression and burnout creeping in. By the time I would recognize it, he said, it would already be too late.

He was telling me that dementia had both of us in its sights; that I had to take care of myself in order to care for my wife.

***

We returned to Kerman, Iran, to be near where we grew up. I continued to read about dementia and plot our course. I joined the international FTD forum and laughed and cried with other caregivers online. The forum was a lifeline, with caregivers sharing ideas and experiences and helping each other find a way forward. More than that, it was a community on a shared journey, of people who understood each other's pain.

And this was not limited to the forum.

After our diagnosis, I wrote to our closest friends to let them know. One of them, a caregiver himself, called to say:

> *I'd offer to help financially, but you don't need my help. I'd offer to help around the house, but you live half a world away. All I can offer is this: when you are at your wits' end and need to scream, call me, and scream at me.*

In Kerman, I set up a caregiving system built around systematic routines and schedules, based on taking data, recording observations, and careful experimentation and continuous improvement. With our days organized around routines, it was possible to sort through clues and get to the bottom of problems when they would inevitably arise. Little by little, our lives began to feel grounded again, and our days became more predictable.

Soon, the phone started to ring. Other caregivers had heard about us from friends and relatives, and sought advice about their patients and their problems. I'll never forget a young man slumped in a chair in our living room, barely eighteen, his face already worn with the weight of dementia. He was asking about his mother grieving and beating herself.

His mother had FTD, too.

His is the other face of dementia: young people at the start of their journey, often women, often the youngest in the family, having to put their dreams on hold in order to care for an ailing parent. Some ten to fifteen years later, when dementia has run its course and caregiving is finally at an end, they find themselves alone and adrift in middle age, with health problems from years of caregiving stress, and without a college education, a career, or a family of their own.

From all these conversations, one thing was painfully clear: the lack of information in Farsi made the difficult task of caring for a loved one with dementia that much harder and more gut-wrenching. To help provide some measure of relief, I set out to write a handful of articles on dementia caregiving and made them available online.

This was the start of the Dardashna Project (literally meaning "One who knows pain"). Along the way I met dedicated medical practitioners and researchers, including faculty members at Kerman Medical Sciences University and Tehran Medical Sciences University. Their support and collaboration helped the project in immeasurable ways, from reviewing Dardashna articles and books, to sponsoring Dardashna in conferences, to offering caregiving courses based on Dardashna material, to disseminating Dardashna books to patients and other practitioners.

Over the past several years, Dardashna has grown to include an extensive website covering all aspects of dementia caregiving, three books published under the sponsorship of Kerman Medical Sciences University, numerous educational clips and podcasts, a forum for Persian-speaking caregivers, and face-to-face caregiver support group meetings.

The book you are reading now is the culmination of this effort, covering all aspects of caring for a loved one during the course of dementia progression, in one place, and in practical, easy-to-understand, step-by-step instructions.

***

I can still remember the bewilderment of the days and weeks following my wife's diagnosis, having to plan a whole new future for both of us, not knowing where to begin or what to tend to first. Despite its warning signs, dementia seems to appear out of nowhere: one day you're living a life that is familiar, and the next day you're facing an immense new obstacle with a steep learning curve. At a time when you're dealing with disorientation, bewilderment, and grief, the last thing you need is to have to go hunting for information across numerous websites and disparate articles just to get a handle on what is to come. A trusted, direct, plain-speaking companion can go a long way toward tamping down anxiety, helping you reorient, and easing you on your way.

It is my hope that the collective wisdom of countless caregivers whose insights are woven into the pages of this book will help make your journey less daunting.

Mehdi Samadani
March 2022

1 | GETTING TO KNOW DEMENTIA

The challenges of dementia are much more manageable once you know how they come about and what they represent. A practical understanding of what is happening helps to make sense of things, and will help focus your efforts where they can have the most impact. It helps you put your loved one's new behavior in perspective, understand how they feel and what they are trying to say or do, and to better help them cope.

WHAT IS DEMENTIA?

By the time my mother was diagnosed with dementia, she had already begun to struggle with depression. We didn't know much about dementia or how we should support her through it. We complained that her cooking had deteriorated and that she was not on top of things as before. This only added to her anxiety and made her depression worse.

Dementia is an umbrella term encompassing a number of progressive brain disorders. Its symptoms include impairment of a wide range of memory and cognitive functions, including remembering, thinking, reasoning, and problem solving. Other symptoms include impairment of language skills, visual perception, self-management, and the ability to focus and pay attention. In the course of dementia progression, major behavioral changes such as mood swings, agitation, depression, and aggression occur with various levels of severity and duration.

Symptoms of Dementia

Memory problems are only one of the symptoms of dementia. They are the most noticeable aspect of Alzheimer's disease, which is the most common form of dementia. Alzheimer's disease accounts for up to 75 percent of all dementia cases in the United States.

While there are many indicators for dementia, at least two types of the following deficiencies must be clearly present in order to suspect dementia as a likely cause:

- The presence of memory problems and forgetfulness
- Inability to communicate clearly
- Inability to follow a conversation
- Inability to focus on tasks involving multiple steps
- Lack of proper judgment in daily affairs
- Improper interpretation of sensory stimuli.

Dementia should not be confused with a general decline in mental capacity due to aging. While it is normal for mental ability to decline with age, such decline is a natural part of aging and has different causes and characteristics than dementia.

She didn't remember how to charge her phone or which way to open the fridge door. She'd get frustrated when she couldn't read the time off of her watch or the clock on the wall. She felt embarrassed at not being able to help around the house and thought she had forgotten how because her family didn't let her do housework anymore.

How Dementia Develops

Dementia is caused by a loss of neurons in the brain, usually over an extended period of time. As losses mount, the functioning of the affected regions grow increasingly impaired, leading to corresponding disruptions in thinking, behavior, and emotional regulation. For example, in Alzheimer's disease, neurons in the hippocampus (the center of memory and learning) are usually the first to be lost. (Figure 1.2) As a result, memory problems are among the first symptoms in Alzheimer's disease.

Different types of dementia begin to take hold in different areas of the brain, but the progressive nature of dementia means that eventually most areas of the brain will be affected. As a result, in later stages of dementia progression, various types of dementia may have very similar sets of symptoms and may appear almost identical. Moreover, symptoms, which are initially isolated and manageable, grow more pronounced and wide-ranging over time, eventually rendering patients completely dependent on their caregivers for even their most basic needs.

The Importance of Timely Diagnosis

Many of the symptoms of dementia are also present in other disorders, including thyroid disease, vitamin deficiency, alcohol dependency, and depression. They may also be due to side effects from medication. Unlike dementia, however, many of these conditions are treatable and reversible if addressed in a timely manner.

Even if the diagnosis turns out to be dementia, timely detection can help keep the condition in check and reduce its rate of progression. Although there currently is no cure for dementia and no way to stop its progression, a lot can be done to reduce its impact on the patient and those around them.

- A range of treatment options is available to help reduce or control some cognitive and behavioral symptoms of dementia, especially during the early stages.

- Early detection gives the patient and loved ones the opportunity to put financial and legal affairs in order, prepare a living will and medical power of attorney, and discuss care options while the patient still has the mental capacity to participate in planning for their own care.

- Most importantly, early detection helps put the care program on the right footing, get everyone to pull in the right direction, and improve quality of life for the patient and their family.

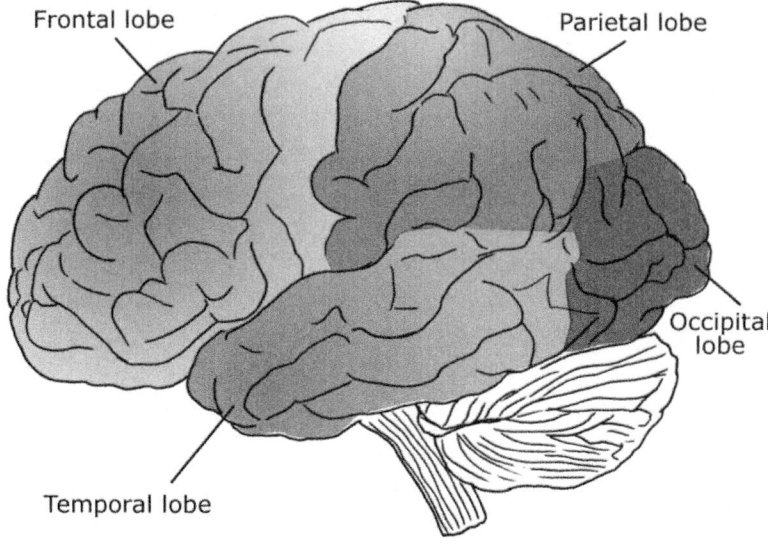

Frontal lobe – higher cognitive functions, including thinking, planning, attention, and short-term memory; aspects of personality, empathy, understanding social cues, and assessing future consequences of actions; coordination of voluntary movements, including speech production.

Parietal lobe – sensory perception, including integrating stimuli from sight, taste, hearing, smell, and touch; body awareness, hand and eye coordination, spatial reasoning, language processing, and writing.

Occipital lobe – vision, including color, distance, size, depth, movement, identifying objects and faces, reading, spatial reasoning, and visual memory.

Temporal lobe – processing affect/emotions, understanding language and speech, and processing certain aspects of visual perception; interacts directly with the limbic system or the "emotional brain," which is key to emotional regulation, memory, and learning.

Figure 1.1 The human brain

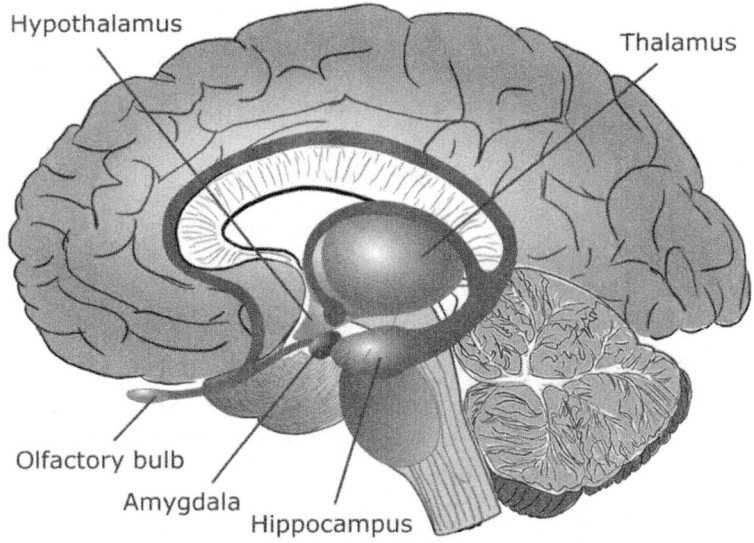

Thalamus – acts as a relay station, passing sensory signals from sensory organs to the associated areas of the brain; regulation of consciousness, sleep, and alertness.

Hypothalamus – regulation of certain metabolic processes, body temperature, hunger, thirst, fatigue, sleep, circadian rhythms, and aspects of parenting and attachment behaviors.

Amygdala – emotional processes, including fear, anxiety, aggression, and the fight or flight response; involved in memory, decision-making, and motivation.

Hippocampus – consolidation of information from short-term memory to long-term memory, spatial memory that enables navigation.

Olfactory bulb – perception of smell; directly projects to specific areas in the amygdala, closely linking the sense of smell with emotions.

Figure 1.2 The limbic system or the "emotional brain"
is key to emotional regulation, memory, and learning.

DEMENTIA WARNING SIGNS

My mother had misplaced her hearing aid. I turned the house upside down trying to find it, looking everywhere she could have hidden it and then forgotten about it. In the evening, my son had just gotten home and had learned about our dilemma. He stood in the middle of the living room for a moment, then went straight to the cupboard in the kitchen, and pulled the hearing aid out of the sugar bowl! Dumbfounded, I asked how he knew where to look. He shrugged, saying, "You searched where things could be hidden. I searched where Grandma visits most during the day. If it hadn't been in the cupboard, my next guess would've been the fridge."

Dementia warning signs have a different flavor than the general decline in cognitive capacity that is a natural consequence of aging. Although the presence of any of these warning signs may not be sufficient grounds to suspect dementia, it is nevertheless recommended that you see your doctor if you or a loved one exhibits one or more of them.

Short-Term Memory Loss

Problems with short-term memory may be an early sign of certain types of dementia. This is different from the typical misplacing of TV remote controls, eyeglasses, or car keys. While misplacing one's glasses may be considered normal, leaving them in the fridge or in a kettle should be considered a warning sign.

At the onset of dementia, short-term memory loss may be quite subtle. The patient may have no trouble recalling memories from a year ago (long-term memory), while still forgetting what they had for lunch earlier in the day (short-term memory). With dementia, short-term memory issues are longer lasting and cannot be resolved by retracing one's steps.

Another early sign of short-term memory problems is when one has trouble remembering what they were doing and why. They might open the fridge door and not remember why they did it. As short-term memory loss gets worse, remembering daily tasks and the order in which to perform them becomes more difficult. It becomes harder to keep track of simple things, like handling eyeglasses while making tea or fishing the milk carton out of the fridge.

Inability to Find the Right Words

Another early sign of dementia is difficulty in expressing one's thoughts. The patient seems to know what they want to say but is unable to articulate it. This hampers their ability to communicate.

It is difficult for a healthy person to fully appreciate that someone with dementia needs more time to search for words, and still more time to express them. As a result, family members may get bored with conversations and avoid interacting with the patient. This leads to the patient becoming increasingly isolated over time, as those around them seem too busy with the bustle of daily life to take the time to engage with them.

Changes in Mood

My mom has become forgetful, but not so much that people outside the family would notice. She keeps asking about the date and the day of the week. She is stressed out, constantly talking about goals and plans that did not materialize. She seems to be suffering from mild depression.

Dementia is often associated with changes in mood and behavior. Depression is a common problem, especially early in the course of dementia progression. For example, 20 to 40 percent of those suffering from Alzheimer's disease also suffer from depression. Although the patient may not be fully aware of the depression closing in, a spouse or children are likely to notice it before long.

Along with changes in mood, the patient's personality may begin to change as well. For example, a person who has been quiet or shy in the past may become highly social and talkative. One reason for such changes in personality is the impairment of judgment and inhibitions. What the patient may have deemed inappropriate in the past may seem quite natural to them now.

Lack of Interest

Other early signs of dementia include lethargy and apathy. The patient no longer shows interest in activities that they used to enjoy. They do not participate in the life going on around them, avoid spending time with friends, and do not get excited by good or bad news anymore. The passing of a loved one, memories of their wedding, or the birth of a grandchild do not seem to have an impact anymore.

These changes are subtle at first and may be dismissed as being caused by fatigue, inadequate sleep, retirement, or old age. However, as these symptoms grow more pronounced over time, they will become quite apparent to the family and will erode the quality of life of everyone involved.

Difficulty Performing Daily Tasks

My mom asked me how the TV works, then watched quietly as I proceeded to explain how the signal comes through the wire and how the TV remote works without any wires. Just then my dad happened to pass by, and Mom asked him the same question. He took the remote control from her and pressed the ON button.

At the onset of dementia, the patient may have difficulty performing daily tasks. For example, choosing the right clothes for work, or selecting clothes that go together, may become difficult. Over time, it becomes impossible to do more difficult tasks, such as keeping track of household expenses or participating in games that involve detailed rules. The patient will have difficulty learning new tasks or following new instructions. For example, they may find it impossible to learn how to use a new cell phone. They may even forget how to do simple things, like using the remote control to turn on the TV.

Confusion

Who is this man who's talking to me? Where is he taking me? What is he asking me?

When one loses their train of thought or forgets a step in a process, it is easy to get lost and not know what to do next. Initially, confusion manifests in the form of lost car keys or misplaced eyeglasses. But over time, it grows and affects daily life in profound ways. Before long, the patient may be unable to recall or articulate words and phrases. They may forget what they were doing or what to do next. They may be unable to remember people's faces, or recognize their spouse or children. They may not remember where they are and may get lost in familiar places, like the neighborhood of their home.

Disorientation

I saw my brother-in-law sitting alone on the grassy median in the middle of a busy street. I pulled over and walked up to him. He recognized me. He said he had stopped at the traffic lights and then couldn't remember where he was or where he was going. All the landmarks, shops, and buildings had suddenly seemed unfamiliar. He assured me that he was okay now, but I could see he was shaken.

Disorientation and lack of familiarity with previously familiar environments are other warning signs of dementia. Disorientation can also manifest as inability to follow instructions. For example, Mom is preparing a meal based on a recipe she has used many times in the past. But she is no longer able to understand the instructions or take the necessary steps in the proper order. The frustration may be enough for her to throw everything on the floor and leave the kitchen in tears.

Disconnect From Events

Mom and I were watching TV the other night, and she couldn't follow the story. She kept asking questions about the characters and why they did this or that. Sometimes when we're talking, she asks a question or says something that has nothing to do with the subject.

Over time, the patient will have more difficulty following conversations or keeping up with the events around them. When there is a conversation going on in their presence, their reactions and general demeanor may seem like they are just a few seconds behind the train of the conversation, never managing to get on board.

This makes it impossible for the patient to participate in everyday conversations, whether at home or at work. Without proper coping strategies, the patient will become increasingly withdrawn and will stop participating in daily activities with the rest of the family.

Often the patient is aware that they have a problem but they hesitate to discuss it with anyone. This may be due to pride, fear of what lies ahead, or worry about how their condition will impact other members of the family. As a result, it is up to the family to notice the warning signs and engage with the patient in order to keep them from further withdrawal and social isolation.

Repetition

What time is it? When is lunch? What day is it? When is lunch? What day is today?

Repeatedly asking the same questions, buying the same thing over and over again, shaving more than once a day, and other repeated behaviors are warning signs of dementia.

It's easy to get frustrated and snap at the repeated questions: "How many times do you have to ask? Don't you remember that I answered this question a minute ago?"

The reality is, they don't. The patient neither remembers the question from a moment ago, nor the answer to it. It doesn't matter how many times they ask and how many times you answer. They cannot form memories of the event. Keeping this simple fact in mind makes it a lot easier to respond appropriately to repeated questions and help a loved one find a foothold in the confusion in which they find themselves every day.

Preferring Routine

People with dementia rely on routines to get by, even in the early stages of their illness. Routines provide continuity through the day and reduce uncertainty and surprises. They channel the events of the day along prescribed and predictable paths, slowing the pace of life a bit so patients can continue to participate and share in it. Over the course of dementia, routines grow in importance, helping to arrange life in ways that make it more tolerable for the patient and manageable for the caregiver.

DEMENTIA PROGRESSION STAGES

Repetition, anxiety, arguments, accusations, aggression, compulsive behaviors, misplacing things, poor eating habits, insomnia, not recognizing their own children or relatives, not recognizing their own home, wandering outside and getting lost, hallucinations and conversations with imaginary people, not recognizing themselves in the mirror, talking to a mirror or arguing with it – these are some of the things that most people with dementia experience at some point.

Dementia symptoms are initially subtle and may go unnoticed even by close family members. But, over time, they become more pronounced and debilitating. Symptoms vary over the course of dementia progression depending on the type of dementia, the part of the brain that is initially affected, and how the damage progresses over time. By knowing the type of dementia and its rate of progression, doctor and caregiver can develop a treatment/care plan to better cope with many of the symptoms and problems that may arise over time.

Caregivers will have questions during the course of dementia progression, such as:

- At what stage of the illness are we?

- How long will this stage last?

- How long will the symptoms last?

- What sorts of complications and symptoms should we expect in the next stage?

Rate of Dementia Progression

It is not easy to estimate how fast dementia will progress in a particular case, or how long it will be before a patient is completely dependent on their caregiver. Sometimes the progression may follow a steady course for a while, even without medication, and then accelerate. In some cases life expectancy may be less than two years after diagnosis, while in other cases dementia may take more than twenty years to run its course.

- Generally, dementia at older ages tends to progress faster, causing older patients to reach the late stage more quickly.

- Other conditions, such as cardiovascular disease, kidney disease, and diabetes are complicating factors and may lead to faster progression.

- Onset, severity, and duration vary from one type of dementia to another. For example, progression tends to be faster in Lewy body dementia than in Alzheimer's disease, while in vascular dementia progression may be slowed or even stopped by bringing risk factors under control.

Stages of Dementia Progression

Doctors use a variety of models to determine the stage of dementia progression for a given patient. These models take into account the patient's physical, mental, and emotional status, as well as the level of care that the patient needs. The most commonly used models divide the course of dementia progression into three, five, or seven stages.

When considering dementia progression models, here are a few things to keep in mind:

- These models are not precise, and the symptoms listed are not the same in all types of dementia. These models should only be used as a guide.

- Symptoms may occur earlier or later than suggested by these models, or may never occur at all.

- Individual capabilities vary among patients and across stages. For example, some patients may be unable to maintain their balance in the middle stage of dementia progression, while others may remain mobile even in the late stage.

- Some symptoms, such as aggression, may occur at one stage and then subside, while others, such as memory loss, may worsen over the course of dementia progression.

The Three-Stage Model

The three-stage model is the most commonly used model of dementia progression and the model used throughout this book. The three-stage model is convenient because of its simplicity and its focus on the progression of dementia after its onset. It divides the course of dementia progression into three stages: the early stage, the middle stage, and the late stage.

The Early Stage

At this stage the patient may be able to live independently, drive, go to work, and engage in social activities. Family and friends may notice problems in some areas, such as in decision-making, but most symptoms go unnoticed by those who do not live with the patient.

Typical early stage problems include:

- Difficulty remembering daily events, people's names, or the right words

- Difficulty performing tasks at work or navigating social settings

- Difficulty in planning, organizing, and decision-making.

The Middle Stage

This is usually the longest stage of dementia progression and may last for years. Over the course of this stage the patient will need increasing levels of help and support. Behavioral changes such as confusion, anxiety, restlessness, and aggression are more pronounced at this stage. Other problems may include:

- Forgetting past personal events, like their wedding date (long-term memory)

- Confusion about time and place, such as not knowing what time it is or where they are

- Needing help in picking out clothes to wear or getting dressed

- Start of incontinence episodes

- Disruption of sleep and waking cycles (circadian rhythms) due to malfunctioning internal clock

- Disorientation and getting lost

- Personality and behavioral changes, including hallucination, suspicion, and repetition.

The Late Stage

At this stage the patient is less aware of the events around them. Speech problems, lack of control of physical movements, and loss of mental and physical abilities necessitate round-the-clock care and support. The late stage is characterized by:

- Need for full-time care, 24/7, and in all matters

- Loss of the ability to walk or sit

- Loss of the ability to speak or communicate
- Eventual loss of the ability to swallow
- Vulnerability to infections and diseases, especially urinary tract infection and pneumonia.

The Five- and Seven-Stage Models

The five- and seven-stage models of dementia progression augment the three-stage model by including pre-dementia phases of cognitive decline as well. These models are mostly used by doctors, due to the models' added focus on the earlier stages of cognitive decline. Although the five- and seven-stage models are not used in this book, it helps to be familiar with them as your doctor may refer to them when communicating with you.

The Five-Stage Model

1. The individual is healthy and does not need any help.
2. Very mild dementia. The individual typically does not need help.
3. Mild dementia. The patient is able to handle daily tasks but may need help occasionally.
4. Medium dementia. The patient needs help with most tasks.
5. Advanced dementia. The patient needs help with all tasks, both physical and cognitive.

The Seven-Stage Model

1. The individual is healthy. No cognitive decline. No dementia.
2. Very little cognitive decline. No dementia.
3. Little cognitive decline. No dementia.
4. Medium cognitive decline. Early stage dementia.
5. Moderate cognitive decline. Middle stage dementia.

6. Moderate-severe cognitive decline. Middle stage dementia.

7. Severe cognitive decline. Late stage dementia.

THE CHANGING CAREGIVER ROLE

Imagine how frightening it is not to be able to remember the names of people you have known for years, not to be able to participate in conversations among your loved ones, not to know why you went to the store or how to get home. Imagine the loneliness of not being able to follow your favorite TV shows with your family, or laugh and cry with them. Imagine being in the dark as to what they're laughing about or why they are upset.

The role of the caregiver evolves during the course of dementia progression. During the early stage, the patient needs love and care, and a family that shows a great deal of understanding and empathy. During the middle stage, the patient's behavioral changes demand a great deal of patience and flexibility from those around them. And during the late stage, the patient's lack of balance, recurring infections, and swallowing problems require great vigilance on the part of their caregiver.

The patient's needs change over time, and the caregiver's role has to adapt accordingly. With advancing dementia, the demands of caregiving grow progressively more complex and may require the support of trained professionals.

The Hardest Stage of Dementia

From the perspective of the caregiver, all three stages of dementia are difficult, each presenting its own set of challenges. From the perspective of the patient, however, the hardest period is the first stage.

It makes the hair stand up on the back of my neck when I think about the early years of my grandfather's illness. No one in the family understood what he was going through. My grandmother kept scolding him to get a grip on his life. Their children joined in on the chorus, telling him to stop being lazy and grumpy all the time. But, what haunts me the most is that he knew he was becoming a burden, and yet, no one seemed to have noticed it when he needed compassion and love the most.

If dementia is a frightening prospect for the family, imagine how it must feel to the patient. Forgetting the names of familiar people and things, not remembering what to do next, or feeling disoriented in your own home can be a source of unbearable anxiety. When holding on to a thought challenges the limits of your cognitive ability and drains all your energy, it's hard to feel like you have any control over what is happening in your life.

Sometimes it is impossible for even the closest family members to appreciate the depth of the patient's suffering. More than at any other time, the patient needs support, empathy, and understanding by those close to them, but family and friends are often in denial. They haven't yet come to terms with the reality of dementia and the patient's new behavior, diminishing cognition, and speech difficulties. Some even seem unable to take any constructive action.

Family members, whom the patient had cared for throughout their lives, now contradict and boss them around constantly. They belittle the patient, scold them like a child, accuse them of laziness, complain that they have grown distracted and grumpy, and demand that they go back to being the person they were in the past.

This can worsen the patient's condition. It drives them away, pushing them further into social isolation and withdrawal, and increases the likelihood that they sink further into depression.

Patient Needs During the Early Stage

The early stage of dementia is sometimes referred to as the post-diagnosis stage. During this time, the patient may experience minor impairment in learning or thinking ability. They can still continue to go to work, participate in daily activities, engage in conversations, eat with others, go shopping, and spend time with family. They are often successful at hiding their symptoms from relatives, friends, neighbors, and even their doctors, and may not seem any different to those who do not live with them. This period may take years.

The role of the caregiver in this stage is that of a partner. During this time, you are a friend, a spouse, or a child who supports the patient. You help them in their daily life and, if necessary, help them plan for the future. It is important that your demeanor and speech be calm and reassuring at all times. Expressions of love and affection, unconditional support, empathy, and understanding are essential comforts for a patient who is beset by anxiety and the unknown on all sides.

Patient Needs During the Middle Stage

My wife believed her hallucinations were real. Everyone kept trying to convince her that she was mistaken, that what she heard and saw was not real. And that made her more agitated. No one understood what she was going through. No one appreciated that what she heard and saw were quite real to her. Instead, we all kept asking "Why did you say that?" or "Why are you lying?"

By the middle stage, damage in the brain has grown more widespread. It is increasingly difficult for the patient to express their thoughts or perform normal daily tasks. They may confuse words, have difficulty dressing, become anxious and angry, and experience a variety of other behavioral changes, including confusion, depression, and hallucination.

The middle stage of dementia progression is usually the longest and can last for years. Incontinence usually starts in this stage, often developing into a full-blown condition during the late stage. By the middle stage, the patient is no longer able to hide their dementia. They realize that they need help but shy away from saying so or are not able to articulate their needs. Family members, for the most part, have come to accept that their loved one's problems are real and serious.

The middle stage demands a lot of flexibility and patience on the part of the caregiver. Over time, the patient's abilities will decline, making the patient increasingly dependent on others. To make life manageable, organize the patient's days around routines. Use daily and weekly schedules to make life more predictable, minimize surprises, and bring some stability to the lives of everyone involved.

Patient Needs During the Late Stage

As dementia advances into the late stage, the patient's care needs grow more complex. Swallowing problems make eating and drinking stressful and time-consuming. Balance problems increase the risk of falls, and ultimately make the patient bedridden. Urinary tract and lung infections are always on the horizon. By this stage, the patient has become completely helpless and dependent on their caregiver for everything. You'll have to keep watch for subtle signs of pain or discomfort, as the patient will not be able to communicate their pain to you.

During this stage, your mission is to maintain the patient's quality of life. Treat them with respect, safeguard their dignity, and generally treat them the way you used to in the past, when they were healthy. Although the patient's ability to speak and express emotions is almost completely impaired, it is still possible to connect with them through physical contact and one-way conversations. Expressions of love and affection, such as caressing the hands and face, hugging, and reassuring words, are effective means of communicating to the patient that they are still loved, cared for, and important.

Is Caring for the Patient Beyond Your Ability?

The care needs of the patient, especially during the late stage, may be beyond what the family is able to provide at home. If you find that it is not possible to care for your loved one at home, do not delay the decision to transfer them to a nursing facility.

Moving to a nursing home or care facility can be done at any time during the course of dementia progression. However, in the early stage when the patient enjoys a higher level of cognitive and physical ability, adjustment to the new environment is easier and the patient is better able to benefit from the social and recreational activities at the facility. In reality, however, most transfers to care facilities take place later than is optimal.

Common Types of Dementia

Currently there are more than 100 types of degenerative brain disorders classified under the general heading of dementia, but only a few types account for more than 90 percent of all cases. Although different types of dementia may have different early symptoms, they all tend to converge in their symptoms as they progress and affect more areas of the brain.

Alzheimer's Disease

Alzheimer's disease is the most common type of dementia and accounts for 60 to 80 percent of all dementia cases. There are more than 5 million Alzheimer's patients in the United States alone. As a result, most research funding for dementia is being channeled into finding a cure for Alzheimer's disease.

Age is the greatest risk factor for Alzheimer's, but an early form, known as early-onset Alzheimer's, can be seen in patients as young as 30 to 60 years old. A common early symptom of Alzheimer's is short-term memory loss. Patients start to have difficulty remembering conversations, people's names, and recent events. Apathy and depression are other early symptoms. Over time, symptoms will include inability to communicate clearly, difficulty in making decisions, confusion of time and place, changes in behavior, and ultimately problems with speech, swallowing, and balance.

Vascular Dementia

Vascular dementia is one of the most common types of dementia after Alzheimer's disease. Vascular dementia sometimes co-occurs with other types of dementia, such as Alzheimer's. However, around 5 to 10 percent of all dementia cases in the United States are due to vascular dementia alone. Vascular dementia is caused by blockage or rupture of cerebral arteries. As a result, cells in the affected area are deprived of oxygen and nutrients, causing them to die.

In this type of dementia, symptoms may appear stepwise and suddenly. For example, a stroke may cause an abrupt loss of mental and physical ability. After a stroke, the patient may not be able to regain their previous levels of cognitive and physical function. If they suffer another stroke, the symptoms, along with the damage, may increase in severity and may spread to new areas.

Strokes do not always present with obvious symptoms like a sudden onset of paralysis. Multiple small strokes may occur without any obvious symptoms, and may go unnoticed by the patient and their family.

Most patients with vascular dementia also suffer from other conditions such as diabetes, high blood pressure, and high cholesterol. Many also smoke.

This type of dementia is more common in advanced age, but there are cases under the age of 60. Symptoms and complications vary from patient to patient. Impairments in judgment or daily decision-making may appear alongside physical complications such as problems walking, or numbness or paralysis on one side of the face or the body. The location of vascular damage in the brain, its severity, and the number of strokes directly impact the patient's level of mental and physical capacity.

Lewy Body Dementia

Lewy body dementia (LBD) is another of the most common types of dementia after Alzheimer's disease. It accounts for about 5 to 10 percent of all dementia cases in the United States.

LBD is more common in older age, but there are cases under the age of 60. Most patients suffer from memory and cognitive problems similar to Alzheimer's. Over time, physical complications and behavior changes develop as well.

LBD has four main clinical features:

- The patient's level of awareness and cognitive function is not stable, varying during the day and in the course of the week. At times the patient appears completely normal, while at other times they may appear highly impaired.

- The presence of visual hallucinations. The patient may see individuals, animals, and objects that are not actually there. They may see, converse, and otherwise interact with relatives who have died years ago.

- The presence of Parkinson's-like symptoms, such as impaired muscle coordination, tremors, and trouble maintaining balance. For this reason, LBD is sometimes misdiagnosed as Parkinson's disease, which is a movement disorder.

- High sensitivity toward certain drugs, especially antipsychotics. Even with very low doses of these drugs, LBD patients may experience side effects that are usually seen in other patients only at relatively high doses of the same drugs.

The pathology in LBD, and the proteins that cause brain cells to die, are also seen in Parkinson's disease. Parkinson's disease is a movement disorder. Patients with Parkinson's may develop dementia toward the late stage of the disease. In contrast, in LBD cognitive problems appear before motor control symptoms develop.

Frontotemporal Dementia

Frontotemporal dementia (FTD) usually occurs between the ages of 50 and 60, but there have been cases as early as age 21 and as late as age 80. Around 60 percent of FTD cases occur between ages 45 and 64, which is the prime age of professional productivity and earning potential. As a result, the financial burden of FTD on families tends to be heavier than other forms of dementia. FTD accounts for about 2 to 5 percent of all dementia cases, but given the increase in research into this type of dementia in recent years, it is likely that this estimate will increase.

FTD is caused by damage to the frontal and temporal lobes of the brain. The frontal lobes are the center of higher cognitive functions such as attention, planning, judgment, and impulse control. The temporal lobes are involved in storing memories, learning, and vocabulary. Together, the frontal and temporal regions mediate various aspects of personality, behavior, decision-making, and speech.

FTD has many subtypes, including the behavior variant and the speech variant. In the behavior variant, patients exhibit behaviors that are completely inconsistent with their personality prior to their illness; in the speech variant, patients exhibit a gradual loss of the ability to speak, read, write, and understand what others are saying.

There are two important differences between FTD and other types of dementia:

- Initial symptoms of FTD usually do not include problems with short-term memory.

- Behavior changes, planning difficulties, and speech disorders tend to appear gradually and over an extended period of time, typically long before a diagnosis of FTD.

Over time, patients lose the ability to plan and organize day-to-day affairs, and keep impulses in check. They engage in inappropriate behavior at work and at home, grow indifferent to personal hygiene, and become highly dependent on their caregivers. Other symptoms include apathy and indifference toward loved ones, obsessive-compulsive behavior, overeating, indulging in sweets, aggression and violence, and a complete loss of reason.

Behavioral and speech changes in FTD can be so severe that they impose a heavier burden on caregivers than Alzheimer's disease. Because FTD occurs at a relatively younger age, when patients are still relatively strong, patients' aggression and violence pose a greater danger to caregivers and others.

The loss of judgment that accompanies FTD often leads to bad decisions, resulting in loss of savings and investments. Due to the decline in planning ability as well as behavioral changes, FTD patients often end up losing their jobs and becoming housebound.

Mixed Dementia

Around 10 percent of people with dementia suffer from more than one type. These cases are referred to as mixed dementia. The most common form of mixed dementia involves the simultaneous presence of Alzheimer's disease and vascular dementia.

Is It Really Dementia?

There currently is no cure for most types of dementia, including those described in the previous section. However, certain types of dementia, and certain disorders that resemble dementia in their symptoms, are treatable. It is important to seek medical diagnosis as soon as possible, since many of these conditions, if left untreated, can progress to the point of no return.

Rapidly Progressive Dementia

Rapidly progressive dementias (RPDs) are rare and difficult to diagnose. They may be caused by a variety of underlying conditions, including neurodegenerative, toxic/metabolic, infectious, autoimmune, and other conditions. Mad cow disease, HIV, hypothyroidism, and vitamin deficiency are some of the conditions that may give rise to RPDs. Unlike most other dementias, the conditions underlying RPDs are, in many cases, treatable. Early diagnosis is critical as RPDs progress rapidly and, if left untreated, can run their course within a few weeks or months. This is in contrast to most other types of dementia, which progress slowly and may take several years to run their course.

Pseudodementia

Pseudodementia is not dementia, in that it is not due to neurological degeneration. Rather, it has its roots in psychiatric disorders that have symptoms similar to dementia. The term "pseudodementia" is often used as a descriptive term for the symptoms associated with depression and other mood-related disorders, especially in advanced age. Unlike dementia, in which the course of the illness is progressive, pseudodementia is potentially reversible by treatment.

- People with pseudodementia are usually fearful of their declining cognitive function, while people with dementia tend to be less concerned about it and may even deny that they have a problem.

- A person with Alzheimer's disease usually has short-term memory problems, while in pseudodementia, usually both short- and long-term memory are impaired.

- Persons with pseudodementia are less cooperative with their doctors and tend to score better on psychiatric tests than expected. In contrast, persons with dementia tend to be more cooperative with their doctors and score lower than expected.

- A patient with pseudodementia is more likely to answer "I don't know" to questions in cognitive tests administered by a doctor.

- Compared to patients with dementia, patients with pseudodementia are better able to focus and pay attention, and rely less on their partners in answering their doctor's questions.

- Many patients with pseudodementia complain about memory loss, but patients with dementia usually do not have this complaint due to their lack of awareness of their impairment.

CAN DEMENTIA BE PREVENTED?

As the exact causes of Alzheimer's disease and most other types of dementia are not yet known, there is no surefire way to prevent them. However, several dementia risk factors have been identified. By implementing effective lifestyle changes, it is possible to reduce the risk of developing dementia by about 40 percent.

Dementia Risk Factors

Age is the most important risk factor for developing dementia, especially in the case of Alzheimer's disease. Various studies have shown a direct correlation between dementia and environmental, disease, lifestyle, and other factors, including:

- Age
- Genetics and heredity
- Lack of physical activity
- Underlying health problems such as cardiovascular disease, high blood pressure, obesity, and diabetes
- Poor nutrition and a diet high in saturated fats, salt, and sugar
- Alcohol abuse
- Mental health problems, social isolation, and depression.

Take Action to Reduce Dementia Risk

Research has identified the following as effective preventive measures against cognitive impairment in old age:

- Education and learning early in life
- Mental activities; increase in cognitive reserve during adulthood
- Healthy lifestyle for cardiovascular health
- Better management of vascular illnesses.

Challenge Your Mind

There is evidence that people who challenge themselves mentally have lower rates of dementia. To keep your mind sharp:

- Read regularly
- Write in a journal
- Take classes and learn new things
- Learn a foreign language
- Listen to classical music
- Play a musical instrument
- Solve puzzles like crosswords and sudoku
- Play strategy games like chess, checkers, backgammon, and Go

- Use your opposite hand to write, and brush your teeth and hair
- Get 8 to 9 hours of sleep at night
- Keep the visual and auditory areas of your brain engaged by checking your vision and hearing every year and correcting them if necessary.

Stay Active

Physical activity increases oxygen supply to the brain as well as the muscles. It not only gets the blood pumping, but also engages much of the brain to affect movement and coordination. It is exercise both for the body and the mind.

- Include cardiovascular exercise such as swimming, walking, and cycling in your daily and weekly schedule.
- Engage in hobbies such as gardening, flower arranging, photography, music, and painting.
- Use meditation and yoga to relax your mind and rejuvenate your body.

Eat Healthy

A low-fat, low-salt diet that is high in fiber, fresh vegetables and fruits, may reduce the risk of Alzheimer's disease and many other types of dementia.

- Enjoy a healthy diet that includes vegetables, legumes, fruits, fish, and olive oil.
- Include nuts and seeds, such as almonds, walnuts, chia seeds, and sesame seeds.
- Avoid saturated fats and processed foods.
- Enjoy sweets in moderation.
- Eliminate sugary drinks from your diet.

Be Social

Research has shown that social people are less likely to develop dementia than those who are isolated.

- Join clubs and participate in group activities and hobbies.
- Join a charity and do volunteer work.
- Engage in group sports such as soccer and basketball.
- Take group vacations.
- Attend gatherings, and visit friends and family.
- Have your meals with friends and family.
- Avoid loneliness.

Reduce the Risk of Vascular Disease

Cardiovascular disease is closely implicated in Alzheimer's disease and vascular dementia. Take steps to improve your cardiovascular health, and reduce your risks of stroke and vascular dementia.

- Quit smoking and other types of tobacco products.
- If you consume alcohol, do so in moderation.
- Eat a healthy diet that includes fresh vegetables and fruits.
- Exercise for at least two and a half hours each week.
- Check your blood pressure periodically and as needed.
- If you have diabetes, follow proper diet and medication.
- Consume salt and sugar in moderation.
- Cardiovascular complications are common after brain injury. Protect your brain by wearing your seatbelt while driving or traveling in a car, and a helmet when skating or riding a bicycle.

2 | FIRST STEPS

A diagnosis of dementia closes one chapter and opens a new one. Now, you have a name for what's been happening and an idea of what lies ahead. But, the story isn't written yet. Now, you have to dream up a whole new future for yourself and the loved one in your care.

It seems daunting at first, and it may take a while to regain your bearings. But once you do, things will begin to feel calmer. With the right plans and routines in place, life can feel grounded again, and the days more predictable. In the meantime, as you stop to catch your breath before pressing on, this chapter offers up a few first steps to help ease you on your way.

Hard days are ahead, but there will be good days, too. Your relationship with your loved one will change, and in the midst of all the challenge and upheaval, there will be moments of connection and love, deeper than any you might have thought possible.

COMING TO TERMS

The first step is to accept that someone you love is ill. If you accept that, you'll find that many of the hardships you'll encounter have a bitter side and a sweet side. In the early and middle stages of dementia, especially, you'll run into issues where you don't know whether to laugh or cry.

Dealing with issues that arise during the early stage of dementia progression requires endless patience and perseverance. Often, the patient insists that they are fine, and may not easily give up control over finances, driving, and other areas of their life. They are usually successful at hiding their symptoms from relatives, who may themselves be in denial about their loved one's illness.

It's Not an Act

She had started sleeping in a different bedroom on a different floor. She had taken her clothes out of the closet and had spread them out, saying it was easier that way. She had moved her makeup desk out of her bedroom and into the hallway. She did things that weren't the results of just forgetting, but seemed more like madness.

The patient may neglect personal hygiene – not wash regularly, skip bathing, and continue to wear soiled clothes and refuse to let you help them change. They may refuse your offer of food, drink, medication, or help with bathroom visits. They may get upset with you, snap at you, or get physical if you insist, or if they believe you are bossing them around.

- Remember that they are not being stubborn or putting on a show. In the face of the overwhelming cognitive effort that it takes to do otherwise, it's just easier for them to say no. Staying thoughtful and considerate is your best chance of getting the patient to eventually cooperate.

Engage With Compassion

It's as if we're dealing with a headstrong child, but one that cannot be taught, one that forgets more each day, one that needs constant monitoring by an experienced and patient grownup. They cannot learn, and yet, as we care for them, all we know how to do is to try to teach... or scold.

Tough love does not work with dementia. You cannot compel the patient to take control of their life or behave the way they used to in the past. This is a time for compassion and understanding, and accepting the reality of their illness.

- Start organizing the patient's life around consistent schedules and predictable routines. The more you can make life simple for the patient, the better they will be able to navigate the challenges of the day, and the longer they will be able to live independently.

- Treat the patient with kindness and respect. Ask them how you can help, and encourage them to share their feelings. Keep them engaged to prevent them from becoming isolated and withdrawn.

- Help them find other patients who are in the early stages of dementia progression. Introduce them to online forums and support groups that specifically deal with dementia from the patient's point of view.

Keep a Daily Log of Events

Slowly she lost the ability to cook: she started making mistakes, then her cooking became simpler, until finally she stopped cooking altogether.

Start a daily log of the patient's condition and activity. Make note of their cognition and physical abilities, as well as all relevant daily events. A daily log can help you monitor the rate of progression of the illness, and provides clues for solving difficult health and behavioral problems down the road.

Join a Support Group

You are not alone. There are communities of caregivers who are facing similar issues. They are valuable sources of information and support. Search for support groups online. Join a forum or two to get a feel for how they work. When you are ready, ask questions, seek advice, and share your experiences with others.

Behavior Problems

Dad wasn't the same person as before. He had become stubborn. He refused to take a bath. Wouldn't show up for appointments. He couldn't concentrate; his mind was all over the place. He had become suspicious of everything and everyone. All his life he had turned the other cheek, but now he was ready for a fight. In the evening, he remembered loved ones and, thinking they had passed away, mourned their passing.

Throughout the course of dementia, especially in the early and middle stages, patients' behavior is a constant challenge and a source of worry and frustration for the caregiver. Still, behavior changes can be managed, usually by identifying and addressing root causes, and without resorting to drugs. You'll have to anticipate issues and redirect the patient's attention with creativity and humor to diffuse difficult situations.

Pilfering

Things would get lost around the house. She kept asking for money, and later, we'd find the money under a rug or stashed in some other corner of the house. One day, relatives came for a visit and, when they were ready to leave, their car keys had gone missing.

Pilfering is a common early problem. The patient may pick up an item from a store shelf and leave without paying for it. They may eat a candy bar off the shelf while they walk around the store, or put something in their pocket and forget about it. This behavior can be highly stressful for the caregiver. It may also lead to conflict with store staff and involvement by law enforcement.

- Do not let the patient go shopping alone. When shopping together, stay with them at all times and keep a close watch.

- At home, keep credit cards, keys, and other small, shiny, or colorful objects out of view. Do not leave candy or sweets within easy reach.

- When something goes missing, approach from the point of view of the item having been misplaced, rather than deliberately hidden. Look in places where the patient frequents, rather than places where they might have hidden something on purpose.

Scolding Strangers

When visiting the park or while shopping, the patient may scold strangers for talking or laughing loudly, admonish mothers to quiet their crying children, or invade other people's conversations. This may be a result of reduced inhibition that has its roots in the destruction of neurons in the prefrontal cortex. Still, the behavior is confusing to others and unnerving for the caregiver who can never be sure how strangers will react.

- Accompany the patient on all their outings. Stay vigilant to prevent such situations from arising in the first place, or keep them from escalating into confrontations.

- Alter your path, distract the patient, or put yourself between the patient and others to minimize the chances of an unpleasant encounter.

- Prepare a small card mentioning the patient's dementia and the possibility of inappropriate behavior. When necessary, hand the card to the other party to prevent an overreaction.

Accusing Others of Theft

After we sold his car, he started accusing his son-in-law of having stolen it.

The patient may stash away items or give items away, and forgetting that they have done so, accuse others of stealing. They may gift a scarf to a relative, and upon seeing her wearing it a few days later, may accuse the recipient of theft and demand the scarf be returned. This behavior is common in dementia and a source of consternation by those who are unaware of the illness and the resulting behavior changes.

- When the patient misplaces an item and accuses someone of theft, do not confirm or deny the alleged theft. You cannot convince them that they are mistaken. Instead, help them find the missing item.

- When the patient demands the return of an item, such as a gifted scarf, return it. Alternatively, avoid the problem by never wearing the item in the presence of the patient.

New Spending Habits

Mom didn't recognize bills anymore. A five-dollar bill and a hundred-dollar bill were the same to her.

Patients often develop a taste for shopping, sometimes buying the same item over and over again. They may purchase common items such as vitamins or toothpaste, stash them in a corner, drawer, or cupboard and then forget about them. Sometimes, patients develop more expensive tastes; they may purchase expensive jewelry and forget about it just as quickly. This behavior is more common in frontotemporal dementia. It may be due to forgetfulness, impaired impulse control, or a compulsive behavior rooted in anxiety.

- Have an ATM card issued in the patient's name, with a limited balance, or a credit card with low credit limit. This way, you can limit the patient's spending, while still respecting their independence.

- Before long, the patient will not be able to tell the difference between a five-dollar bill and a hundred-dollar bill. If the patient wants to hold on to cash, give them cash in small bills.

My wife had developed a taste for jewelry. She had bought a couple of smaller pieces already, then had promptly forgotten about them. This time, she had her eyes on a not-so-small necklace. Betty, the clerk at the jewelry counter, sensing something was not quite right, leaned in and gently said, "This will be on sale next week. Buy it next week." I'm not sure how much of that registered with my wife. But Betty saved us on that day.

A couple days later, my wife wanted to go to the mall again. Despite my best efforts, we ended up at the same store. She peeked around to the jewelry counter and started waving me in. "Betty is not there," she said. "Hurry, before she gets back!" Before I knew it, she had handed her credit card to the cashier.

HOME AND MEDICATION SAFETY

For a long time, I hesitated to encroach on Mom's personal space. But, over time, our definition of personal space had to change. First it was financial affairs, and the freedom to spend her own money, that had to go. Then it was shopping and the freedom to leave the house alone. Then interaction with friends and relatives had to be regulated. And then household chores, like cooking and cleaning, went off-limits. Within three to four years, all she was able to do on her own was to eat, wash, or go to the bathroom.

Medication Safety

Find a way to take over the responsibility of managing the patient's medications for them. They may resist, insisting that they can do it on their own. However, it won't be long before they start making mistakes about the timing or the dosage of their meds. They may miss a dose, take it twice, or mistake their meds for food or candy and take a large amount in a short period of time.

Home Safety

Patients will gradually forget how to properly use or handle household appliances and chemicals, or even what purpose they serve. They may turn on the gas to the stove, but forget to light it, or they may use a spoon to stir a blender while it's running. Due to an impaired sense of taste and smell, they may drink liquid detergents, or cook with bleach or other household chemicals.

- Put dangerous items and materials out of reach of the patient.

- If the patient smokes, stay with them while they do it. A lit cigarette or pipe is a fire hazard.

- Do not leave the patient alone. Shadow them wherever they go and keep a watchful eye for potential hazards.

Getting Lost

One day, he got lost on his way to work. For 24 hours we didn't know where he was or what had become of him. Then, someone called. Alerted by my dad's incoherent speech, they had recognized that there was a problem.

Dementia patients may forget where they are or where they were going. They can wander outside their home and get lost in their local neighborhood. Wandering and getting lost is a serious risk for patients who are mobile and have memory impairment.

- Do not let the patient go out alone. When outside, do not let them out of your sight. You may have to hold hands to make sure that they don't wander off during a brief moment when you are distracted.

- Write down the patient's home address and phone number on a small card. Include a few words about their dementia and any other relevant conditions, such as diabetes. Laminate the card and put one copy in the patient's purse or wallet and another in their jacket pocket, where it can easily be found by the police or others trying to help the patient find a safe return home.

Finding Strength in Vulnerability

> *Coming home early one day, I ran into an old acquaintance of my wife's in our driveway. As we exchanged pleasantries, I noticed she was holding a nice purse, like the one my wife had. She seemed uncomfortable and anxious to get going, so it was a short conversation. Inside, I noticed an old worn-out purse on the sofa. I asked my wife about it. She said that she and her old "friend" had exchanged purses on her way out!*
>
> *A couple of weeks later, I was picking up my wife from the hairdresser's. As I helped her into the passenger seat, I glanced over to make sure she had her purse with her. Just then, I saw a young woman rushing toward us. She was holding something gingerly between her fingers. "I think your wife made a mistake," she said, trying to hand me a crisp hundred-dollar bill. "This is too much tip." It was all I could do to keep myself together long enough to mouth the words: "No mistake! She wants you to have it."*

To walk with dementia is to know vulnerability. Sometimes it may feel like the firm ground is giving way under your feet. What you used to take for granted turns into unexpected sources of vulnerability, and what you never counted on in the past turns into welcomed sources of support and strength. Accepting vulnerability means thinking ahead of new risks and working out how to reduce or eliminate them. It also means being open to sources of help and support that are out there, waiting to be discovered.

- Awareness is the first step to empowerment. Just knowing to look for pitfalls on the path goes a long way in helping you to avoid them.

- Remind yourself not to get complacent. Continually reevaluate your routines to make sure they are still safe.

- Think outside of the box to identify new and unexpected vulnerabilities, and to find ways to reduce or eliminate them.

- Do not dwell on vulnerabilities as negatives to be lamented. Instead, approach them rationally: identify problems, then figure out how to fix them.

- Take care of your emotional health. A mind burdened with stress and grief cannot stay vigilant, consider all options, or predict and solve problems before they arise.

FINANCIAL, LEGAL, MEDICAL

He signed on to a number of bad deals that eventually cost him his business. He bought fancy brand-new tires for a car he had sold years ago. Little by little, he stopped paying rent and utilities. He didn't pick up after himself, didn't do chores, didn't pick up trash lying around the house. He'd collect discarded food from a public trash bin to feed birds in our back yard.

Safeguard Finances

Some patients may still be able to work for some time, especially if they own the business. But, due to impaired decision-making, they may make poor financial or legal decisions. They may give away large sums of money to strangers, bankrupt a family business, or lose a lifetime of savings at a stroke of a pen. At home, they may be enticed by TV ads to buy items they don't need, or fall prey to phone and online scams.

Put Legal Affairs in Order

Take care of financial and legal matters and discuss the patient's future care while they still have the ability to participate in the decision-making process.

- Discuss with the patient their care preferences, especially as it relates to issues arising in the late stage of dementia progression. Do they wish their life to be prolonged through artificial means, such as ventilators and tube feeding, if the need should arise?

- Prepare a durable power of attorney (DPOA) and a healthcare directive, preferably with the help of an elder care attorney.

- If the patient wishes to make a will, or change an existing one, this is the time to do it. To minimize any future issues, all these preparations should be completed and properly documented with the help of an elder care attorney.

Attend to Postponed Medical Procedures

If the patient needs medical procedures that have been postponed for one reason or another, this is the time to attend to them. This includes dental work, and adjustments to dentures, prescription eyeglasses, and hearing aids. Tend to these and other medical needs early, while the patient still has the ability to understand and cooperate with you and their doctor. This window of opportunity is short-lived and will close rapidly.

- Managing swallowing problems is one of the primary challenges during later stages of dementia progression. If the patient has swallowing issues now, consult with a speech therapist.

Address Addiction

If the patient suffers from addiction or other substance abuse problems, seek guidance from specialists with expertise in both addiction and dementia. Depending on the specifics of your situation, your doctor may recommend addiction treatment or strategies to help you manage the patient's addiction through the course of dementia progression.

Driving

> *Soon, she started having trouble on the road. It was like she didn't notice road signs anymore. One time, she slammed on the brakes, thinking there was a ditch in front of her car. On the highway, when a car would pass her in the adjacent lane, she'd brake, thinking it was her car that was moving backward.*

Whether the patient should continue to drive or hang up their car keys is a common area of contention during the early stage of dementia progression. Patients often insist on driving well past the time when it is safe for them to do so. According to the National Institute of Health, nearly one fifth of patients with documented dementia continue to drive, and two-thirds of those who continue to drive have impaired driving ability.

Signs of Unsafe Driving

- Forgets addresses, gets lost in familiar places.
- Lacks awareness of time and place.
- Does not pay attention to road signs.
- Does not observe speed limits.
- Drives slowly and makes mistakes.
- Gets brake and gas pedals confused.
- Becomes angry and confused while driving.
- Does not pay attention to street curbs.
- Has frequent car accidents.

How to Ask a Loved One Not to Drive

She thought she was lucky in finding a parking spot whenever she needed one. When her car got towed, we found out that she had been parking in front of fire hydrants.

Ideally, you want to get the patient to agree to stop driving. This is likely an anxiety-provoking subject for the patient, as it would mean giving up a large measure of their independence. By addressing their anxiety, you're more likely to get them to cooperate. If unsuccessful, however, you may have to resort to more extreme measures, such as hiding the car keys, disabling the car, or selling it.

Getting Help From Your Doctor

In many states, doctors are required by law to report to the local health department if a patient is diagnosed with dementia, or is impaired in a way that makes them unable to drive safely.

- Ask your doctor to advise the patient not to drive anymore. Patients usually respect their doctor's advice more than that of their spouse or caregiver. Make sure to get the doctor's order in writing so you can show it to the patient if they forget.

Getting Help From the DMV

In many states, you can request the Department of Motor Vehicles (DMV) to evaluate the driving skills and safety of a loved one that you deem unsafe. You can request the DMV to not divulge your identity. Based on the results of a road test, restrictions may be placed on the driver, like not being able to drive at night, during rush hours, or on freeways.

- If the patient's driver's license is revoked, you can direct the blame at the DMV. This may help to redirect the patient's anger and get them to cooperate with you.

Notify Your Insurance Company

I asked my wife to pull over for a minute while I ran to the store to pick up our order. As I was waiting to pay the cashier, I looked over and saw my wife standing next to me. Surprised, I asked if she had found a parking spot. "No," she said. She seemed so calm, so innocent, that I panicked. I ran outside and found the car double-parked, driver's door ajar, with the engine still running.

People with dementia are advised to contact their car insurance carriers to ensure that their insurance policies remain in force. Amendments may be required to cover for their illness. Insurance companies may refuse to pay damages if a person with dementia gets into a car accident and the company was not informed of the dementia at the time of diagnosis.

TRAVEL

Right away, she lost her passport and wasn't even concerned about it. While on the trip, wherever we went, she thought she had already been there. She thought she knew people she had never met and would start conversations with strangers. She didn't remember if she had had lunch, or whether it was day or night.

Traveling is still possible in the early and middle stages of dementia progression, but with proper planning and lots of precautions. Whether it is advisable to travel is a question that requires careful weighing of the benefits against the risks involved.

Traveling is stressful for a person with dementia, and their reaction to the added stress can be unpredictable. The changes in their daily routine, the unfamiliar environment, and the pace of activities all add to the confusion, anxiety, and aggression that the patient experiences in the best of times.

Plan for Travel

- If possible, travel with a trusted person who can assist you during unexpected events or situations. Expect that the patient's behavior will be much more problematic while traveling than on a regular day at home.

- Make a list of everything that you will need ahead of time so you don't forget anything important. Take extra clothing for cold or warm weather. Pack ample incontinence supplies, wet wipes, snacks, and drinks. Include slippers and neck pillow for additional comfort. Provision for the patient's entertainment on the way, including music, storybooks, photo albums, and so on.

- Take along medications, medication list, dosage and time instructions, your doctor's phone number, and other essential and emergency phone numbers.

- If you plan to fly, ask your doctor to write a letter indicating the patient's type of illness and their special needs, and requesting help and cooperation, especially from airport security staff and flight crew.

- Think through possible incontinence scenarios, such as in the departure area or on the plane. How would you deal with them should they arise?

While on a Trip

- Do not pack too much into a day. Plan more time than usual for every activity. Allow plenty of time to rest and recharge between activities.

- Try to make the patient's daily schedule during the trip resemble their regular schedule at home as much as possible.

- Prepare for the possibility of wandering. The patient may get disoriented in unfamiliar environments, wander off, and get lost. Stay with the patient at all times, and do not let them out of your sight.

- Be ready to pick up and return home on short notice. Your trip may need to be shortened unexpectedly due to unforeseen circumstances.

When Visiting Family and Friends

Although the patient may not remember the names of friends and relatives, they will enjoy seeing familiar and friendly faces. When planning to visit friends and relatives, alert your hosts about the patient's special needs ahead of time so your hosts can better accommodate the patient during their visit.

- Stay calm in the event of mishaps. Treat the patient with respect at all times.

- Do not address the patient like you would a child. Avoid baby talk and any other speech or behavior that could be demeaning to the patient.

- Do not discuss the patient's illness or behavior in front of them.

- Ask friends and relatives to stay in the patient's field of view. Have them approach gently, smile and make eye contact, introduce themselves, and call the patient by name to draw their attention.

- Ask everyone to respect the patient's personal space and not get too close unless invited to do so by the patient.

- Encourage people to use hand and face gestures when interacting with the patient for better communication.

- Make certain that your host does not offer any food or snacks to the patient before consulting with you.

- Use a photo album or a puzzle to keep the patient from getting bored.

- If the patient starts to get upset, change the subject to distract the patient.

- Be prepared to terminate your visit and leave abruptly, if necessary.

CHILDREN AND DEMENTIA

When a loved one is afflicted with dementia, the lives of close family members undergo profound changes. The upheaval in the family and the associated stress and exhaustion create an environment where the needs of other vulnerable family members may go unmet. Children are especially vulnerable to the toxic effects of chronic stress and grief in the family, and require extra care and attention.

Talking to Children

A close encounter with dementia can trigger a flood of emotions in children: distress at the prospect of losing someone close to them, fear that other loved ones or themselves will fall victim to dementia, and guilt that they are the cause of their loved one's illness.

- Explain to children that their loved one's behavior changes and speech impairment are not on purpose, or directed at them, and are caused by dementia.

- Ask how they feel about their loved one's illness. Listen carefully to their answers to learn about their concerns and fears. Provide comfort and reassurance accordingly.

- Adjust your explanations to the children's age, maturity, and tolerance levels. Answer their questions clearly and truthfully. Assure them that you are ready to answer any other questions that they may have, now or in the future.

- Some children may hide their distress and unhappiness, and pretend to be unaffected by their loved one's illness. Talk to them about their feelings and what's going on in the family, while respecting their way of dealing with the situation.

- Teenagers may seem preoccupied with their own affairs and spend more time in their own rooms, alone. This may be a defense mechanism in the face of intractable problems of dementia. While respecting their privacy, assure them that you love them and they can talk to you if they want, at any time.

- Encourage children to keep a diary. Writing about their feelings can be therapeutic and can help them organize their thoughts and sort out their feelings.

Shielding Children

In some circumstances, children may have to assume responsibilities that are usually handled by adults, such as shopping, cleaning, or cooking. They might even take on some of the caregiving duties. This premature adulthood is deeply damaging to a developing child, and may lead to frustration, resentment, depression, and other problems.

- Let children help in caregiving tasks, but take care to let them have their childhood. Children need to play, study, and enjoy life in spite of the struggles of the family.

- Be mindful of how you carry yourself in front of children. Children learn how to deal with the pain and anxiety of living with dementia by observing how adults react to these challenges.

- Assure children that, in spite of all the pressures and caregiving duties, you love them the same as before. Make plans to spend quality time with them on a regular basis.

If a Child Has Difficulty Coping

Watch for signs that a child is having trouble coping. Dementia forces children to confront emotional challenges that can grow overwhelming over time. Pay attention to chronic feelings of:

- Grief about what has happened to someone they love

- Anxiety about what will happen to their loved one

- Frustration at the patient's repeated questions and stories

- Embarrassment at their loved one's strange behaviors in front of their friends

- Confusion over changing roles: having to care for someone who used to care for them

- Despair that all the efforts expended in caring for their loved one is in vain

- Anger that their parents are busy caring for someone else and cannot spend enough time with them.

If a child acts up, has disturbing dreams, or complains about a vague pain, they may be suffering from anxiety disorder. Other warning signs include having difficulty concentrating in school, and poor or deteriorating academic performance. If necessary, inform their school counselor about dementia in the family.

Grandpa can't go out anymore. We have to lock the doors to keep him from getting lost outside. When he walks, we have to hold him so he doesn't fall, and when it's time to sleep or wake up, we have to help him lie down or get up. Sometimes he gets so upset that he cries really hard. He thinks people on TV are real, but he doesn't recognize himself in the mirror. He doesn't remember my name, but he still remembers me. When we visit him and I hold his hand, he caresses my hand. When we say goodbye, he kisses my cheeks. When I put my head on his lap, he strokes my hair.

3 | Planning for Effective Care

Arguably, the best place to care for a loved one with dementia is at home, provided that it can be done effectively. To be viable, your home care plan must include a dementia-friendly home, a primary caregiver who has the trust and support of the rest of the family, and sufficient resources to fund the care process for the long haul.

- Consider any stairs, ease of access to the bathroom and shower, and the level of noise and activity at home, including the presence of young children. Is the home environment suitable for providing care into the future?

- Do you have the necessary help to care for the patient day in and day out, indefinitely? Understand that promises of help by friends and family may not materialize into action.

- Are there daycare facilities nearby? Is it possible to drop off the patient at these facilities on certain days of the week so you can have a few hours to rest or tend to other tasks?

- Do you have the necessary funds at your disposal to hire someone to help out as dementia progresses and care needs grow more challenging?

Physical limitations of the living environment may make it impossible to care for the patient at home, especially during the middle and late stages of dementia progression when the patient becomes wheelchair bound and their care needs grow more complex. However, it is often human-related factors and family dynamics that are among the most difficult issues complicating the care process, especially early on.

GETTING EVERYONE TO PULL TOGETHER

Once dementia appears on the horizon, there is a short window of opportunity to address important questions about the future, progression of dementia, care plans, financial and legal affairs, and so on. Care issues will only grow more challenging over time, and it is important to get the care effort going in the right direction from the very beginning or as early as possible.

Dealing With Denial

My dad was in denial about my mom's illness. He believed that her behavior was deliberate, like she was playing a role. He blamed himself for having focused so much on work and career, instead of tending to her emotional well-being. As Mom grew more dependent and aggressive, Dad grew more frustrated, scolding the children for encouraging Mom's shenanigans. This went on until he learned more about dementia. Now, he is much more helpful and constructive, but he feels guilty for how he treated Mom early on. The other day I caught him weeping. I now have both parents to worry about.

Often the first roadblock to establishing a care program is denial. The patient's spouse, children, relatives, or friends may refuse to accept a diagnosis of dementia and rationalize the patient's difficulties as being due to fatigue, depression, or natural aging. They may even accuse a member of the family of having caused the problems by stifling or coddling the patient.

Denial is common in early stages of dementia when the symptoms are sporadic and even members of the immediate family are not aware of all of them. It won't be long, however, before they recognize the scope of the problem and come to terms with the diagnosis. Still, some may stay in denial for months or years.

Unfortunately, a person in denial is unable to meaningfully participate in the care planning of a loved one, and may even be unable to engage in a constructive way. In the meantime, dementia continues its progress regardless of whether everyone accepts the reality of the situation, or whether they start to make plans to deal with it.

Bringing Everyone up to Speed

My aunt has two very sensitive adult children who haven't been told about their mother's dementia diagnosis. I'm concerned that the news may be distressing to them, and yet, I need to find a way to ease them into knowing what is coming, help them accept their mother's illness, and guide them through the necessary steps to deal with it.

Have all the stakeholders on board from the beginning. Family members, close friends, and relatives should have full knowledge of the patient's dementia and its ramifications. They should know what to expect, so as not to be embarrassed by the patient's behavior when it inevitably deviates from what is considered "normal." Most importantly, family members should learn as much as possible about dementia so they can help their loved one cope, rather than aggravate their condition.

Dealing With Disagreements

Slowly I learned that my wife cannot change back to who she was and that I am the one who has to adapt to our new reality. I learned to be selective about the gatherings that we attended, and to avoid folks who have no clue about dementia and no inclination to learn about it. That's how we became lonelier over time, but our life became more tranquil.

In some cases, care planning is straightforward. If you are caring for your spouse, are physically and mentally healthy, have the necessary financial means, and enjoy the unconditional support of your children, then managing the care process is relatively straightforward. You can make all the decisions with the sole focus on what is best for the patient, without having to worry about approval or interference from others.

Often, however, things are not that simple. Even close family members do not always arrive at the same conclusion at the same time. They may disagree about the nature of the problem or how best to go about solving it. Sometimes, family members might put up obstacles, rather than participate constructively. When planning for care, it is important to address interpersonal issues early on and continue on an ongoing basis.

- When planning your care strategy, have a meeting with all the stakeholders present. Discuss caregiving and related issues, including legal, financial, management, and follow-through of the plans over time. Try to reach consensus among all the parties.

- Don't assume that everyone is on the same page regarding care planning and decisions. Most likely, you'll find that various members of the family have different ideas and disagree on the correct approach. Discuss the issues early on and try to reach an agreement so everyone is on the same page, supports the plan, and works toward its success.

- Past grudges among family members may make it impossible for everyone to get along. Some members of the family may constantly create problems and find faults with others, without providing any help themselves. Sometimes, the best thing to do is to let them get it off their chest and then move on with the real work of planning.

- If there are many disagreements and deep family grudges going back many years, especially among the primary family members, it may help to have a neutral body, such as the family attorney or a counselor, present during these meetings.

PRIMARY CAREGIVER AT THE HELM

The primary caregiver is the most critical element of a successful care program and the primary pillar on which everything else rests. The primary caregiver must not only do most of the heavy lifting in day-to-day care of the patient, but must also take on a leadership role, directing all aspects of the care program, including marshalling financial and human resources of the family to get the job done.

The leadership role, however, is often overlooked, especially when it falls on a younger member of the family to take on the role of the primary caregiver. In family dynamics where everyone thinks that they're in charge and that the primary caregiver is simply there to follow instructions, there is a real danger that the patient will not have the benefit of a primary caregiver who can take ownership of the difficult task at hand.

Choosing the Primary Caregiver

> *Everyone said that I was making a big deal over nothing, that she was just tired, depressed, or in need of a vacation.*

The most natural choice for the role of the primary caregiver is usually the patient's spouse. Often, however, the spouse is unable to take on that role due to denial, illness, physical and other age-related issues, or lacking in energy or organizational skills necessary to do the job. In these situations, it often falls on the children, usually the youngest daughter, to care for the ailing parent.

- When choosing a primary caregiver, consider their other responsibilities, such as continuing education, career, family and children, physical and mental health, readiness to take on the task, and interest in doing so. If the primary caregiver's workload does not allow them to manage the care duties on a dedicated basis, they may not be the best choice for the job.

- If the caregiver is a younger member of the family, such as a son, a daughter, or an in-law, will the spouse, siblings, or relatives let the primary caregiver manage the care process on their own? Or will they disrupt the care process with criticisms and other interference that will get in the way of providing care to the patient?

- Is the caregiver realistic when it comes to issues of care? Do they approach the situation from a systematic, problem-solving point of view? Do they accept that the patient has dementia, or are they in denial, believing that the patient is just being difficult or stubborn? Do they treat the patient with empathy and understanding, or do they believe that being strict will help the patient snap out of their condition?

- Is the caregiver able, physically, mentally, and emotionally, to manage the caregiving responsibilities?

KEEPING THE CARE PROCESS ON COURSE

An essential task of the primary caregiver is to keep the care process on track and under control. The care process must remain stable, yet flexible and evolving. Decision-making and planning must be adjusted over time to fit the evolving needs of the patient. At the same time, schedules and routines must remain consistent, and not fluctuate in response to opinions of those who are not intimately involved in the care process or lacking the necessary experience.

Accepting Advice and Criticism

My siblings don't help in caring for our mom. I am the sole caregiver and under a lot of pressure. No one helps, but everyone is ready to point out faults with how I do things. They criticize in ways that show they don't understand the issues, and yet, they're all too busy with their own lives to want to try and learn for themselves.

Well-meaning advice from those not involved in day-to-day care often turns out to be wrong. When you receive advice from acquaintances, carefully consider the advice. Use your experience and judgment to decide which to adopt and which to ignore.

- If you are not the primary caregiver, leave the daily decision-making to the person who is. Timely and thoughtful suggestions are welcomed, but unnecessary criticism and fault finding serve only to discourage and demoralize the caregiver. Recognize that it's the primary caregiver who is living with the patient, is deeply involved with their day-to-day care, and is intimately familiar with their care needs.

- If you are the primary caregiver, be open to suggestions and invite others to share their ideas. Even if not quite on the mark, suggestions can help as a springboard to other ideas that can work. Take suggestions in the spirit intended, even if the manner in which they are offered leaves something to be desired.

There may be times when there's no choice but to listen to baseless criticisms from one person or another. The best solution is usually to just listen, then continue with your care plan. The primary caregiver has no choice but to continue to provide care for the patient, and the more conflict that can be avoided or sidestepped, the better.

Managing Visitor-Patient Interactions

My father's tremors have worsened since his mom's passing. A relative, offering condolences, told him, "Your mother died because she couldn't bear to see you sick. You must feel guilty now, even though you don't show it."

Even well-meaning sentiments, when expressed thoughtlessly, can cause a lot of harm. Providing care often involves teaching others about the patient's condition, and what may or may not be said or done in their presence.

- Consider writing a couple of pages of instructions for close friends and relatives, with a few words describing dementia, and explaining how to behave in the presence of the patient.

- Let everyone know that large family visits are not appropriate given the patient's condition. Ask parents to not bring noisy children when they come to visit.

- When someone negative is visiting, stay with the patient and try to control the theme and direction of the conversation.

- Limit contact between the patient and troublesome individuals. In extreme cases, you might have to consider cutting off contact between such an individual and the patient altogether.

Staying in Control

I'm fortunate to have a caregiving system that enjoys a lot of privileges, for which I am grateful. I know of many caregivers who manage with a lot less. Having the benefit of these privileges, the care process is a lot more manageable and predictable at our home:

My wife and I are the only people living in our home.
I enjoy relatively good health.
I know what is to come and I prepare for it.
I know that my wife is not being stubborn.
I'm not jealous that my wife has a caregiver.
Family visits to our home are limited and controlled.
No relative is allowed to interfere in our care process.
I have the full support of our children in the decision-making of the care process.
I manage behavior problems using care-based interventions.
I have help from dutiful and well-trained caregiving aides.

FINANCIAL AND LEGAL PLANNING

With advancing dementia, different patients exhibit different rates of decline across the spectrum of cognitive and decision-making functions. Given this uncertainty, it is critical to put the patient's finances and legal affairs in order as early as possible, before they can do irreparable damage to their financial health. This also helps to ensure that their decisions cannot be challenged in court on the grounds of having been made with a legally unsound mind.

Safeguarding Finances Early On

> *My husband was recently diagnosed with frontotemporal dementia. For months I've been concerned about his work. He has a consulting business and works alone supporting his clients. Over the past couple of years, his performance has deteriorated significantly. He can't focus on anything for more than a few minutes, doesn't answer emails, and doesn't seem motivated to finish anything anymore. He has lost most of his clients already. Those that remain complain that their problems go unresolved for long periods of time.*

Patients will ultimately develop difficulty in financial decision-making, and may end up squandering their life savings or running a family business into the ground. Bad investments, buying or selling things, or helping others financially beyond their means are some of the common ways in which patients drain their life savings. With their nest egg ruined, it becomes very difficult to provide adequate care for them over the course of their illness.

- Choose a trusted person to take over the management of the patient's financial affairs early on. Consult a family attorney and take care of the necessary legal paperwork so your financial designate can take over when it's time to do so.

- The financial designate will be responsible for handling all financial affairs of the patient, including paying the utility bills, rent and property taxes, household expenses including food and groceries, and doctors' fees and other medical expenses.

Managing Finances for the Long Run

Caregiving expenses tend to rise during the course of dementia progression. It may become necessary to procure a wheelchair and a hospital bed, make modifications to the patient's home, or hire additional help. If expenses exceed the patient's income and savings, you'll have to find ways to make up the difference.

- Make a plan for all the expenses ahead of time to ensure that the care program will proceed uninterrupted. Make sure that income and expenses are balanced before you run into a problem and have to scramble for a solution that, by then, may be out of reach.

- If you are not able to afford the financial costs, what are your fallback plans? Are there others who will be able to help with the expenses?

- Those who undertake to pay part of these expenses must be clearly identified. The timing of the payments, the amounts, and how they will be paid must be agreed upon and documented.

- Individuals providing financial assistance must fulfill their obligations on time to eliminate the need for follow-ups by the caregiver or the financial designate.

- If the available funds do not meet the projected expenses, you must reexamine your proposed care plan. Adjust as necessary until your care plan and the available resources are balanced to your satisfaction.

Putting Legal Affairs in Order

Mom and I had gone out to file some papers. I filled out a form and then asked her to sign it. She stared at me. I asked again, "Sign here, Mom," but she seemed even more confused. I asked if she remembered how to sign her name, and she didn't respond. At home the next day, she remembered. We've been practicing together since then, but her signatures don't always match.

For a transaction to be legal, the persons making the transaction must be of a sound mind. For a person with dementia, soundness of mind can be challenged in court, especially since there are no clear and accepted metrics to define when the mind becomes legally unsound.

That's why it is important to put the patient's finances and legal affairs in order as early as possible. Prepare the necessary legal documents, preferably in consultation with an elder care attorney from their state of residence. Among the essential legal documents are a durable power of attorney (DPOA) and a healthcare directive.

- A DPOA is a legal document giving a person whom the patient trusts the authority to manage their financial affairs. DPOAs remain in force even when the patient is incapacitated.

- A healthcare directive is a legal document that allows the patient to express their wishes regarding their future healthcare, medical care, and end-of-life decisions, when they are no longer able to make those decisions.

Patient's Wishes Regarding Their Own Care

Early on, when the patient is still able to participate in decisions regarding their own care, the family should sit down with the patient and try to understand their wishes. Take clear notes of these discussions to avoid misunderstandings in the future. Consult an elder care attorney to make sure decisions cannot be legally challenged.

- Who should take over the patient's financial and legal affairs, and when?

- Is the list of the patient's assets and liabilities up-to-date, properly documented, and kept in a safe place?

- Has the patient prepared any wills and testaments? Are they current? Does the patient wish to make a new will and testament?

- What are the patient's wishes for their medical and nursing care? In case of incapacity or when necessary, where and how should their care be provided? Who should make care decisions for the patient?

- Who should participate in end-of-life decisions? How should those decisions be made?

- What are the patient's views on quality of life? How should it be evaluated?

End-of-life questions, including life support, tube feeding, and quality of life decisions are very difficult, especially for patients and families who do not have direct experience with end-of-life situations. For help, consult end-of-life and palliative care specialists, psychologists and psychiatrists, or religious counselors.

GUARDING AGAINST ABUSE

The relationship between patient and caregiver is based on trust and relies on a caregiver's commitment that is stable, enduring, and unconditional. People with dementia are especially dependent on that trust and particularly vulnerable if that trust is violated. Cognitive problems make it hard for others to decipher if a patient's complaints are real or imagined. Speech problems may make it impossible for the patient to ask for help. Consequently, abuse may go on for a long time, subjecting a vulnerable patient to physical and emotional harm from which they may not be able to escape.

Types of Abuse

Some types of abuse are obvious. Most people wouldn't dream of engaging in physical or sexual abuse of a loved one in their care. Other types of abuse may creep in over time due to frustration and caregiver burnout. Even the most well-meaning caregiver may not always be aware when they get close to the line.

Examples of abuse include:

- Hitting, biting, pushing, shaking, kicking, burning, slapping

- Inappropriate touching, unwanted sexual contact, sexual harassment

- Mocking, humiliation, disrespect, isolation; threatening and other speech or behavior that causes fear, anxiety, and nervousness

- Neglect in providing care, inadequate or improper nutrition, not paying attention to the health and hygiene of the patient, not visiting a doctor when needed, and neglect in routine daily care

- Denying the patient the use of conveniences such as telephone, television, and the use of their funds or other property in ways that negatively affect their quality of life

- Stealing money; unauthorized or improper use of the patient's property for the benefit of someone other than the patient.

Signs of Abuse

Victims of abuse are often embarrassed to admit that they have been abused. They may worry that if they complain, the abuse will get worse. Most dementia patients are unable to complain or otherwise report if they have been subjected to abuse. It is therefore up to you to watch for signs of abuse and investigate if the patient:

- Seems depressed, confused, anxious, or withdrawn

- Has difficulty sleeping

- Shows signs of trauma, for example, rocking back and forth

- Is isolated from family and friends

- Is not interested in activities that they used to enjoy

- Has unexplained wounds, injuries, burns, or scars

- Appears underfed or dehydrated; has unexplained weight loss

- Is over- or under-medicated; not receiving proper medical care

- Appears dirty, not bathed, or is wearing dirty clothes

- Has bedsores and other preventable conditions.

Caregiver Stress and Patient Abuse

Caring for a person with dementia is a labor of love and can be highly rewarding. It is also very hard and stressful. Providing nonstop care, 24/7, is exhausting. Preparing meals, providing daily care, personal hygiene, bathing, grooming, dressing, feeding, and administering medications is a never-ending reality for many caregivers who do not have an adequate support structure to lean on.

Caregiver burnout is common and is a major concern. It harms the caregiver and deprives the patient of adequate care. Under the persistent weight of exhaustion, grief, and depression, the caregiver may neglect to provide care for the patient, without realizing it. In some cases, the caregiver may even abuse the patient verbally and physically.

Caring for the caregiver is a responsibility for the whole family. The caregiver is bearing the brunt of the load of caring for a loved one with dementia on behalf of the rest of the family. If the caregiver buckles under the pressure, the whole caregiving process will unravel.

Whey my mom got sick, my younger brother who was living with her said he'd take care of her. She constantly complained about him, accusing him of theft. She complained that she'd go to sleep with her money under her pillow, and when she'd wake up, the money would be gone. My brother denied it, and we believed him.

She complained that he'd take the batteries out of the remote control that we had installed to help her manage the lights. He denied it. And we believed him. One day, I opened the remote to show my mom that she was mistaken. To my surprise, the batteries were missing! I closed the remote again, and put it back where I had found it. When my brother came home, Mom accused him again, and he denied it again. Then he went to the other room and brought the remote and handed it to me, to prove he was telling the truth. Surprise, surprise: the batteries had reappeared!

Mom heard voices at night, and we thought she was having hallucinations. My brother swore there was no one there. It turns out that he was telling the truth. There were no strangers in the house. Only he would talk from the other room in voices, making like there were strangers there having a conversation. We confronted him, and he said it was a joke. He promised he wouldn't do it again. And we believed him.

Eventually, Mom became bedridden. She had bedsores on her body. We'd treat one side, and more would appear on her other side. Sometimes, she'd go limp, like she was in a coma. It finally dawned on us that he had been drugging her.

4 | GETTING HELP

Dementia caregiving is not a one-person job. It is impossible to care for a patient all by yourself, day in and day out, indefinitely. Providing care for the long haul requires help and support from many people, including hired aides, family members, and friends and acquaintances. It is your job as the primary caregiver to lead others, to invite them to participate in helpful ways, and to delegate some of the hard work of providing care to willing partners.

MAKE IT EASY TO RECEIVE HELP

> *I am the only girl in the family. I have two brothers who can't do the washing and bathing of our mother. It's been four years that she is bedridden. I am 55 years old, and I find it extremely difficult to tend to my husband and our children, in addition to caring for my mom. I have severe pain in my back and both arms. I don't know how to ask for help.*

Remember that as the primary caregiver, you are the person with the clearest understanding of the care issues at hand and the needs of your patient. You are also the best judge of where you need help and when you can accept it. Many friends and family members may want to help, but they don't know what help you need or how to offer it. It is up to you to ask for help and tell them exactly how they can help.

- When asking for help, express your specific need clearly. Give it some thought beforehand so you can properly articulate what you need, when, and how.

- Keep a list of tasks that you can delegate to others. When someone does offer to help, you'll be able to help them help you in a meaningful way.

- Be mindful of your helper's fitness. Do not ask for help from a friend who is tired or sick. Either ask someone else or wait for a more appropriate time.

Ask the Right People for Help

Different members of the family often do not have the same attitude toward patient care. Some may want to control every detail, while others just talk, make promises, but do not deliver. Some only criticize and blame others for everything. In some cases, previous feuds between family members may make coordination and cooperation with the parties impossible.

- Do not ask for help from someone who is unable or unwilling to give it. Do not argue or fight about help that will never come. Accept reality and move on.

- Do not engage with negative friends and relatives. They will not contribute, and they will sap your energy. Remember, you'll need every ounce of your energy to care for your loved one.

- Writing off a negative individual frees you from expectations. It also reduces involvement, interference, and criticisms from someone who is unable to take on a more constructive role.

- Rely on individuals who are willing and able to help, and make the best use of their help. Keep your eyes on the main goal, which is providing care for a loved one who needs you.

Match Tasks to Abilities and Interests

Even family members and close friends living far away can participate in caring for a loved one in substantial and meaningful ways. It's often just a matter of putting the pieces of the puzzle together.

- A neighbor may be able to help mow the lawn or help with grocery shopping.

- A friend may be able to take the patient for a walk in the park.

- A family member who enjoys cooking can help in the kitchen.

- An acquaintance who likes to drive can take you and the patient to the doctor.

- A youngster can keep company with the patient and read to them.

- A sibling who lives far away can call regularly and have a heart-to-heart with a brother or sister who is the primary caregiver.

Divide Tasks Into Coherent Groups

Allow each person to take on a related set of tasks so they can learn the nuances and develop expertise in their respective areas of responsibility. This makes it a lot easier for everyone to do their tasks quickly and reliably, and with less acrimony and with fewer errors.

- Task one person with medical affairs, such as making doctor's appointments, and purchasing and organizing medications.

- Leave the responsibility of taking the patient to the doctor with the primary caregiver. It is the primary caregiver who has the most detailed knowledge of the patient's condition and is the best person to answer the doctor's questions.

- Task another person with financial and legal affairs, such as paying bills, filing and paying taxes, and raising additional funds from members of the family if necessary.

- One person may take on the responsibility for construction, modification, and repair issues around the house, such as building ramps, installing safety grab bars, or doing the necessary modifications to the bathrooms.

- Another person may take charge of shopping and food preparation.

Commit to Consistent Schedules

Keep commitments and schedules consistent. Agree to have the shopping done on specific days and at specific times. Commit to take over, or hand over, caregiving responsibilities according to a prearranged schedule, say from 2:00 to 6:00 pm on Mondays and Thursdays. Consistent schedules enable both parties to plan ahead, meet their obligations, and take full advantage of the time available.

- Do not make a commitment if you cannot keep it.

- Keep commitments sacred. Show up on time, every time.

- Do not cancel or shift commitments around unless there is a real emergency.

Keep Everyone in the Loop

Provide adequate and up-to-date information to all those who are involved in the care of the patient. Keep everyone informed of all care-related events so they can pick up where another has left off, if the need should ever arise.

- Keep a daily log of events as they relate to patient care, to be reviewed regularly by everyone involved in the care process so everyone is up to speed at all times. (See Chapter 6 for more on this.)

- Schedule periodic meetings with family members and friends who are involved in the care process. Discuss all relevant issues, including dementia progression, tasks completed and pending, and any issues with which you are grappling.

- Discuss your mental and physical status honestly. If you do not speak up, others may remain in the dark, believing that everything is under control.

SUBSTITUTE FOR THE PRIMARY CAREGIVER

People's lack of knowledge about dementia and how to care for the patient makes the job harder for the caregiver. There is a lack of cooperation and support from family members. Everything falls on the shoulders of one person. Everyone expects that the main caregiver should never get bored, angry, or depressed, and should never complain.

Caring for a loved one with dementia is hard work. It is impossible to truly grasp the extent of the physical and psychological burden on the caregiver, unless one has experienced it firsthand. Only someone who has walked a mile in their shoes can fathom the extent of the workload and how hard it is to carry it out day in and day out.

- Experience caring for a loved one with dementia firsthand. Take over the role of the primary caregiver for a week or two to give the main caregiver a chance to rest and recover.

- A sibling may plan to fly in and take care of a parent for one or two weeks each year so their brother or sister can take a couple of weeks off for respite or to go away on a vacation.

Taking over the task of caring for a loved one for a week or two gives one an opportunity to engage with dementia and its workload. It's a chance to gain a deeper understanding of what is involved, and get a better appreciation of the effort and its burden. It can bring loved ones closer to each other, and to the patient, and foster deeper bonds among the family members sharing the workload. Most importantly, it helps the primary caregiver stay healthy longer so they can continue to do the vital work of providing round-the-clock care for the patient, while others are busy with their own lives, families, and careers.

Don't Get in the Way of Care

If you are not the main caregiver and cannot offer help, then at least don't get in the way of the care being provided. Remember that sniping at the person providing care, even if only to aggravate someone you dislike, will only get in the way of the care being provided to someone you love.

- Keep the big picture in mind. A healthy caregiver who feels the love and support of the family is better able to provide care for a loved one. An unhealthy caregiver, aggrieved and distracted by unkind words, will not be able to provide the best care possible.

- Don't forget to give the person providing the lion's share of the care a hug and words of encouragement and support at every opportunity. Express appreciation and gratitude for the important work they have undertaken, partly on your behalf.

PROFESSIONAL SERVICES

My grandmother has dementia, and my mom has been taking care of her. My mom has her own health issues and can get agitated by my grandmother's behavioral problems. This in turn agitates Grandma, who starts to cry, swear, and hit herself. The commotion spills over to my dad, who intervenes by cursing them both.

In the early and middle stages of dementia progression, help from friends and family can go a long way in making care at home practical. They can help by taking over shopping, cooking, cleaning, and providing company for the patient when you are busy with something else or need some personal time off.

In later stages, however, you'll usually need additional help and more specialized services. When you notice this need on the horizon, raise it with others in the family right away so you can discuss and reach a consensus well ahead of time.

Adult Daycare Centers

Senior centers or adult daycare centers are resources you can rely on to care for the patient for a few hours during the day, while you tend to other tasks or get some much-needed rest. These centers usually have regular group activities, and may provide personal care, nutrition, and medication administration.

- Initially, the patient may not feel comfortable going to such facilities. This reluctance is usually short-lived, and the patient adjusts to the new environment quickly, and looks forward to going there again.

- To make the patient interested initially, you can suggest that they go there to help others. Once the ice is broken, they will likely want to go every day and stay as long as possible.

- Before deciding to leave the patient in the care of a center, investigate the center thoroughly. Evaluate their group programs, the quality of services, nutrition, staff, and so on. Ask for references and talk to families who have used the services before. Find out how satisfied they were and if they would recommend the center to you.

- After deciding to rely on a care center, continue to stay involved. Visit the center regularly to ensure that the quality of the services remains satisfactory.

Home Care Providers

If you need to hire staff to help care for the patient at home, a service provider company can help you with the process. These companies usually have a standard contract; they provide the workforce and in exchange receive a finder's fee and/or a monthly commission.

- Before signing a contract, have your family lawyer review it and make sure that your interests are protected.

- Make sure that the service provider company does a thorough background check of any candidates that they introduce to you.

Service companies are convenient in that they introduce you to candidates; if you are not satisfied with a candidate, the company will send someone else. Keep in mind, however, that changing caregivers is stressful for both you and the patient. Training a new aide in your care routine, daily schedule, nutrition and medication regimen, and so on will be time consuming – and your responsibility.

Professional Nursing Services

When you need professional nursing care, like administering injections and bedsore treatment, call a professional nursing service provider and ask for the specific services that you need. The services may be offered on a per-call, hourly, or 24/7 basis.

HIRING AND TRAINING

If you find someone to help you care for your loved one, if you find someone who is careful, conscientious, caring and compassionate, if they care for yours as if caring for their own, know that you have struck gold. Treat them with utmost care. Make every effort to look after them in turn as they look after your loved one, and by extension, you.

Another way to meet the increasing demands of caregiving is to hire the help you need directly. The process is similar to hiring a service provider company, except that you'll also be taking on the upfront work of advertising for candidates, fielding calls, and weeding through applicants. If you're up to the challenge of handling the entire process from advertising to signing a contract, you can forgo the help and expense of a service provider and search for help on your own.

Many of the steps are similar to those involved in dealing with a service company, and whichever way you choose to go, much of the work of writing job descriptions, selecting and training aides, and supervising them will remain on your shoulders.

Although direct recruitment is a time-consuming task, it can be made easier with proper planning and a methodical approach.

Look for Local Applicants

- Put flyers on community bulletin boards in shopping centers, churches, gyms, and community centers close to your home, or buy ads in local newspapers and Penny Savers.

- Specify your home's general whereabouts so you attract locals. Applicants who have a long commute to get to your home may be motivated at first, but will lose interest as time goes on and the long commute begins to wear on them.

Keep the Interview Process Organized

- Decide on the specifics ahead of time, such as working hours, job description and responsibilities, educational background, experience requirements, and pay rates.

- Have one person handle all calls from applicants to ensure communication consistency. Use a phone interview to weed out applicants and save everyone's time when a match is not likely.

- Invite promising candidates for a face-to-face interview, preferably at the patient's residence. Discuss the workplace, type of services required, hours and days, time off, and other relevant issues.

- Keep careful notes about applicants' personal information, experience, references, and so on. With multiple applicants and interviews, you are bound to lose track of such details quickly.

Finding suitable help is not easy. First, you have to consider the patient's personality and find someone that they like and approve of. Then, you have to make sure the candidate understands that they are not dealing with a "normal" person and must be prepared to deal with issues that are unique to dementia.

Do Your Due Diligence

Remember that you are inviting this person into the inner sanctum of your home and entrusting them with the care of someone extremely vulnerable. As much as you may be eager to get started, do not lose sight of the fact that a bad match can be a lot harder to undo than you might expect.

- Ask the applicants about their previous work experience. Ask for references and contact them to get their views about the applicants and their abilities, personality, and work ethic.

- When you find a suitable applicant, do a background check to make sure everything is as it appears and there are no hidden issues or unpleasant surprises down the road.

Prepare and Sign a Formal Contract

- Write up a job description and go through it in detail with the candidate. Discuss work hours, what needs to be done for and with the patient, any cooking or cleaning, and so on. This job description must be flexible so it can be updated as needed over time.

- With the help of your legal advisor, prepare a contract spelling out working conditions, responsibilities, compensation, justified and unjustified absences, the existence of a monitoring device such as a closed-circuit television (CCTV), and so on.

- Have the contract signed by both you and the applicant, and witnessed by at least one impartial body, before having the applicant come to work.

Train the New Staff Properly

I had hired a new aide to help care for my mom, had trained her for a few hours, and then left her alone with my mom for a couple hours. By the time I got back, she had packed up and was quitting. She complained that my mom was difficult, had scolded her for changing into something more comfortable, and had demanded, "Who are you?" and "What are you doing in my home?"

The training period for a new aide will vary according to the complexity of the work. Caregiving is delicate work and learning to do it safely cannot be rushed. Take the time to make sure the new aide learns the nuances of care, such as the intricacies of how to handle, move, and feed the patient.

- Before you leave a new aide alone with your loved one, make sure that they know what their duties are and can perform them well.

- Train the new aide in emergency procedures, such as falls and fires. Periodically review the procedures with everyone to make sure they know what to do in case of an emergency.

Provide Clear Supervision

An experienced aide understands the caregiving needs of dementia patients and is familiar with most of the issues that are part and parcel of this condition. However, even experienced staff need proper supervision to make sure that everyone is pulling in the same direction and everything is done according to the broader roadmap.

- Have a single person in charge of supervision and management of hired staff. Do not let friends and family members bombard a new aide with a request here and a critique there.

- Let everyone know that all suggestions or comments regarding the care process should go through a single individual tasked with supervision and management of the hired staff.

Stay Vigilant

- Use closed-circuit television (CCTV) in the rooms frequented by the patient and the aides. Let the new aide know that you have a monitoring system installed, and preferably, state this fact in their contract. Unfortunately, patient abuse is a reality and people with dementia may be unable to report such cases to anyone.

- Keep expensive items, jewelry, and cash in a secure place. This will help give you peace of mind, and reduce anxiety and unwarranted suspicion.

My wife and I have been fortunate to have the help and support of dedicated caregiving aides, and I have been sorry to see them go one by one, each time they had to move to a new city, get married, or otherwise get on with the next phase of their lives. It's hard watching them say goodbye to my wife and see her lose a little more of life with each farewell. It's hard not to get attached, or worry about them as they navigate their own lives, as if they were your own children.

And then the unthinkable happened. One aide borrowed my wife's jewelry and refused to return it. She demanded cash, too, lots of it, or else she would have me beaten or accused of impropriety. It was all so inexplicable. She had been kind, careful, and conscientious, the kind of person you could trust with a vulnerable loved one and your home. And suddenly, she was a different person, the kind that would plant a recording device near your wife's bed, hoping to get some dirt that she could use later.

It was months before life would get back to normal. There were meetings with the police, attorneys, and court hearings. There were changing of the locks, installing security cameras around the house, strategizing about what to do in case of assault by one of her boyfriends, and relatives standing watch when I'd be helping my wife into and out of the car at night. There were sleepless nights, feelings of embarrassment and betrayal, and wondering if there had been warning signs that I had missed.

I still don't know what brought this on, only that she had been inspired by bad movies, worse friends, and tales of con artists seducing and then extorting older men. I cringe to think how vulnerable we must have seemed for a spark so dim to have lit the fuse on such an outlandish scheme.

PLANNING FOR CARE AT A NURSING HOME

My dad and I care for my mom who suffers from dementia, and my brother who has a psychological disorder. Caring for two patients at home with different needs is beyond our ability. We can't separate them from each other, and we're all constantly at each other's throat. My dad is not well, and the situation is wearing on him. I'm really worried about his health.

There may come a time when the patient's care needs surpass what can realistically be provided at home. Care needs grow more complex over time. Recurring infections, lack of balance, swallowing problems and the associated dangers of choking and aspiration pneumonia demand increasingly specialized skills from the caregiver. Eventually, the patient will need round-the-clock care, seven days a week. If the care needed is beyond the ability of the family, placement at a nursing home may be the best and only option.

- When planning your care strategy, consider that the road ahead will be very long, possibly spanning many years. Is the family able to provide all the care that will be needed indefinitely?

- Remember that the care process grows more complex over time. Do you have the skill set necessary to provide adequate care at home, all the way to the end?

- Is the family emotionally and physically able to handle the caregiving challenges into the future, or are family members already exhausted from the demands of caregiving?

- Are caregivers able to meet their other family responsibilities, such as caring for young children?

- Is the health of the patient, or that of their caregiver, at risk?

- Is the social environment of a nursing home more suitable for the patient than their home environment?

- Consider the layout of your home and the special equipment that you'll need, such as a hospital bed, hoist, wheelchair, and so on. Is it practical to care for the patient at home?

Moving a loved one to a nursing home is usually a difficult decision and quite painful for the family. Often, family members oppose this option because they cannot bear the thought that they are somehow abandoning their loved one. Such feelings of guilt and shame are common, and can be very strong. They are, however, not a justification against nursing home placement.

The primary concern should always be the comfort and safety of the patient and whether their care needs can be met at home. Equally important is keeping the patient happy, safeguarding their rights as an individual, and treating them with the dignity and respect they deserve. These kinds of issues must be considered with an open mind, and the golden rule should be meeting the needs of, and providing the best possible care for, the patient.

How to Evaluate a Nursing Home

Care facilities vary in the services that they provide. The quality of care, the ratio of patients to caregivers, group and recreational activities, the types of patients and their illnesses, as well as nutrition, medical care, and cost vary from one nursing home to another. Sifting through all these variables may take a while. It is best to start the process early so you don't have to scramble to find a care facility when the need arises.

- If you believe that you'll need the services of a nursing home in the future, do not delay your research. Some nursing homes have long waiting lists, and if you leave it to the last minute, you might not be able to get your loved one into the residence of your choice.

- Research the nursing homes in your area. Evaluate the costs and the type and quality of services they provide. Learn about their care routines and staff, and whether you'll have easy access to their management.

- Before signing a contract, be sure to visit their facilities several times to see them in action and ensure that the quality of care and programs on offer are according to your expectations.

- Participate in their group activities, such as painting, music, dance, and storytelling, to experience them firsthand. See if the staff makes an effort to include all the residents in the activities.

- Ask the management of the care facility for references. Consult with other families who have placed loved ones at that residence. Ask them about their experience and their satisfaction with the services provided.

- The best option is a care facility that offers the services you want, at the quality you desire, within your budget, and close to where you live so friends and relatives can visit your loved one easily. You might not be able to get everything you want, but you can try to optimize your selection given your specific situation.

When It's Time to Move In

Contrary to popular belief, most patients get used to the new environment very quickly. They may object to the placement at first and cry and beg you to take them home. Be patient and allow your loved one to adjust to the new environment. You may be advised by the staff at the nursing home to avoid visiting your loved one for one or two weeks so they can adjust to the new situation.

- Help your loved one adjust by decorating their room at the nursing home with familiar items, such as their favorite furniture, dresser, pictures and paintings.

- Experience has shown that patients usually have a better quality of life at a nursing home where they can interact with others who have similar issues and can participate in recreational and group activities that are tailored to their condition.

- If your loved one is in the early stages of dementia progression, they are better able to adjust to the new environment and take advantage of the amenities available there.

Facing the Guilt and Shame Afterwards

After five years of caring for my mother at home, I put her in a nursing facility. It was a hard decision, but I just didn't have the strength to continue caring for her at home. There was a lot of conflict with my dad, who could not tolerate my mom's behavioral changes. And I have two young children that need my attention. Still, I can't help but feel guilty, and our relatives are only too happy to pile on.

Shortly after placing your loved one in a nursing home, you will likely struggle with the decision you have made. Did I do the right thing? Did I abandon my mother? Was this the best decision? Should I have given it more time to sort itself out? Was there something else I could have done instead?

There will be a lot of guilt and doubt, and you should be mentally prepared for it. Do not second-guess your decision. Remind yourself that you made the decision with the best interests of your loved one at heart, and that sometimes placement in a nursing home is the best option for the patient as well as their caregiver. Feeling guilty and ashamed is natural, but you should not let it take over your thoughts.

Another reason why you should rein in feelings of guilt and shame is that you'll probably get enough of it from some relatives. Sometimes, people who lack intimate knowledge of your situation will criticize your decisions. Remember that this was and remains a family decision, and relatives and acquaintances have no right to interfere.

Caring for the Long Haul

Nursing home placement is the start of a new chapter in the care process. Your caregiving role and responsibilities do not end; they just take on a new form. With the nursing home now providing ongoing and professional care for your loved one, you get a chance to spend more quality time with them.

You are now your loved one's advocate at the care facility and must continue to oversee their care and tend to their affairs. You may visit your loved one regularly, walk with them on the nursing home grounds, and help them eat. You'll need to stay informed about their condition, behavioral changes, medications, exercise, leisure and recreation, and every other element of their care.

Many caregivers go to the nursing home every day. They feed their loved one themselves, walk with them or push their wheelchair, and participate in group activities with them. They keep a vigilant eye on how their loved one is being cared for at the residence, and make sure their rights and wishes are fully respected.

DEALING WITH CRITICS

A few days after placing my mom in a residence, a distant relative called. This was the second time in as many years she had called to ask about my mom. "Where's your mom?" she asked. I told her we had placed her in a care facility because caring for her at home had become impossible. She started crying, and said, "Why did you abandon her?" I tried to explain, but she abruptly said goodbye and hung up.

In the course of caring for a loved one with dementia, you will come across people who are unable to look past how they feel to grasp the reality that you and your loved one face day in and day out. A person whose reaction is entirely self-focused is unable to see what you need, and wholly incapable of providing any meaningful help or support.

When you care for a loved one with dementia, it is painfully obvious how their awareness of the world around them is shrinking, as if a light illuminating their surrounding is dimming a little more each day. Dementia brings home the fact that our awareness has limits. We live inside our own bubbles, limited by our light and how far it shines. And sometimes, it doesn't shine very far.

That's why you shouldn't put much stock in what people say or how they judge your situation. It's pointless to fault people for not seeing past their light, or fret over their words when they cannot see.

So, the next time a perennial critic calls, feel free to not answer the phone, or say that your loved one is receiving the best care possible. If they still don't get it, tell them it's a private family matter and none of their business.

5 | DEMENTIA–FRIENDLY HOME

The home environment can be a source of major hazards for a person living with dementia. Stairs and uneven surfaces, toilets and bathrooms, kitchen appliances and stoves, inadequate lighting, small rugs, slippery surfaces, children's toys, clutter, and so on represent potential hazards, chief among them, the risk of falls and fractures.

Early in the course of dementia, survey your home for safety and patient comfort. Group home-improvement tasks into coherent sets, and tend to them in order so by the time care needs grow to a particular level, the required amenities are in place.

STAIRS, RAMPS, AND ACCESS

I used to barricade the stairs to the second floor with dining room chairs so I'd be alerted if my wife wanted to venture upstairs. One day, things were quiet for a while, so I peeked around the hallway to the stairs to make sure everything was alright. There was no sign of my wife. At the foot of the stairs, my barricade had been breached and, all the way at the top of the stairs, stood a solitary dining room chair. It hadn't occurred to her to just put the chair aside; she had taken it with her, step by step, all the way to the top.

During the early and middle stages of dementia, when the patient is able to move about, ensuring patient safety can be especially challenging. Starting in the middle stage and into the late stage, ensuring wheelchair access to important areas such as bathrooms may need special planning.

It is important to assess your home early on, and plan any construction or alterations as soon as possible. The risks of falls and other accidents are present from the very beginning and only increase with time. Likewise, access and usability taken for granted today may not remain so for long. Although the patient may not need an access ramp just yet, it won't be long before a ramp will be easier to climb than steps, and much safer.

If You Live in a Two-Story Home

One of the most popular story configurations for a residence is the two-story home, where the living spaces (kitchen, living room, etc.) are on the primary floor, and bedrooms and main bathrooms are upstairs. Unfortunately, the second floor will quickly grow inaccessible, even dangerous, for a patient with dementia.

- If you live in a two-story home where the patient's bedroom is upstairs, move their bedroom downstairs as soon as possible.

- If the main bathrooms are located upstairs, you'll need to make arrangements for when the patient is unable to walk or stand on their own, putting the upstairs bathrooms out of reach.

- If you are considering installing a lift, be sure to consider all of the patient's future needs, including wheelchair access and a hospital bed.

Stairs and Steps

Evaluate stairs and uneven surfaces and install the necessary safety measures to ensure safe and easy access.

- Keep the stairs leading to the upper floor and the basement off-limits to the patient. Take whatever steps necessary to prevent the patient from venturing upstairs, or down to the basement.

- In the early stage of dementia, the patient may be able to negotiate a few steps at a time, such as entrance steps to their home. Soon, however, the patient will find it hard, and ultimately impossible, to climb even a few steps.

- Use anti-slip tape on steps to reduce the risk of slips and falls. Choose a tape with color that is different from the color of the steps so the patient can see the tape more easily.

- Install handrails to help the patient feel more secure and stable as they climb steps.

Access Ramps

Eventually, even a couple of steps will turn into an insurmountable barrier. Access ramps are the most practical way to negotiate barriers, even before the patient is completely wheelchair bound.

- Do not postpone building access ramps until you are out of options. Access ramps should be ready for use the first time you need them.

- Building an access ramp involves competent planning, with attention to factors such as slope, width, material, construction, standard practices, and legal requirements. Consult a competent building company for more information.

- Construct access ramps for critical areas that are accessible by one or two steps, such as the entrance to the patient's home.

- Make sure the ramp has a slope that is gentle enough so a caregiver can easily manage a wheelchair, with the patient sitting in it, both up and down the ramp.

- In the United States, the Americans with Disabilities Act (ADA) requires that ramps that serve public areas have a slope of at most 1:12, or at most 1 foot rise for each 12 feet of horizontal run. In certain cases, a ramp may be as steep as 1:8, or at most 1 foot rise for each 8 feet of horizontal run.

Although the ADA regulations are directed at areas designed for public accommodations, the standards also serve as a useful starting point when planning private amenities, such as ramps for your home.

Walkways and Hallways

Inspect the areas frequently used by the patient and remove furniture, children's toys, and any other items that may trip the patient or otherwise create a fall hazard.

- Small rugs, especially on ceramic tiles or slippery floors, can slip and cause the patient to fall. Either remove such rugs or fix them firmly in place.

- The edges of carpeting, uneven floors, and bases of doorframes extending above the floor are potential stumbling blocks and fall hazards.

- Use colored tape on hallway floor and walls to help point the patient in the direction of the bathroom or their bedroom.

- Put a photo or a nametag on doors to various rooms, such as the bathroom and the kitchen, to indicate the room's purpose. Put the sign at a level that is in the patient's field of view.

Doorways and Wheelchairs

Eventually, transporting the patient from one room to another, including to the bathroom, will require the use of a wheelchair. Make sure the critical areas of your home are wheelchair accessible, long before the need arises.

- Measure the width of the doorway to the bathroom and make sure it is wide enough to allow a wheelchair to go through.

- Sometimes, removing a door altogether may provide the extra one or two inches necessary to allow a wheelchair to fit through.

- Make sure the doorway is wide enough for the particular wheelchair that you have, or will be using. Verify that this is true for all the wheelchairs you'll be using, including a bathroom wheelchair.

- Manual wheelchairs are equipped with hand-rims attached to the rear wheels so a user can propel the wheelchair. Since the patient will not be able to use the hand-rims, you can remove them to make the wheelchair narrower by about two inches. This may be enough for the wheelchair to fit through narrower doorways.

Door Handles, Latches, and Locks

During the early and into the middle stage of dementia progression, when the patient is still mobile, you'll need to take extra precautions to keep the patient inside where they should be, and out of where they shouldn't be.

- Prevent accidental wandering and getting lost. Lock any door that leads to the outside, including the front, garage, and backyard doors. Hide the keys or put them out of easy reach. Install bells or electronic alert systems on exit doors so you are alerted if they are opened.

- Make sure the patient cannot lock themselves inside the bathroom, bedroom, or other areas at home. The patient may lock the door from the inside and not remember how to unlock it. If the latch or lock cannot be opened from the outside, remove it completely.

- Lock the stairway to the basement. If possible, make the stairway to the second floor inaccessible.

- Lever door handles are easier to use, while round doorknobs are harder to grip and turn. Equip doors with lever handles to make access easier for the patient. To prevent access, choose round doorknobs, or remove door handles altogether.

SAFE BATHROOM

In most homes the space allocated to bathrooms is relatively small, making it hard for the patient and caregiver to both fit in, and maneuver, in the confined space. Furthermore, the walls and floors of bathrooms are usually covered by hard materials, such as ceramic tiles. As a result, the risks of falls and injury are greater in bathrooms, and extricating someone after a fall is more difficult.

Toilet Safety

- Raise the height of the toilet seat to make it easier for the patient to sit down and get up.

- Install a toilet seat with a different color than the bathroom walls and the floor so it is easier to see. Alternatively, you can use brightly colored tape to make the toilet seat stand out against its surroundings. When the patient can see the toilet seat clearly, they feel more secure trying to sit down.

- Equip the toilet with backrest and armrests to reduce the risks of the patient falling. You can purchase toilet safety frames separately and install them on existing toilets.

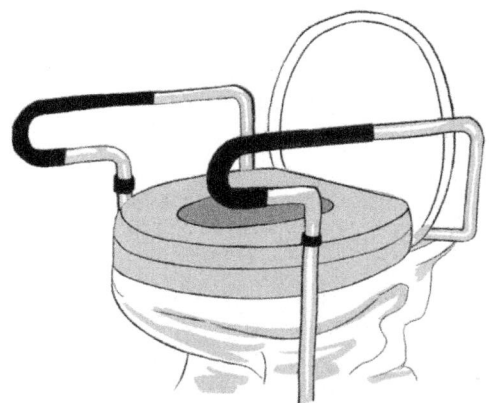

Figure 5.1 Toilet with raised seat and safety rails.
Choose a seat with contrasting color so it is easier to see.

Portable Toilet

- To reduce the need to walk to the bathroom in the middle of the night, put a medical commode or a bathroom wheelchair in the patient's bedroom. If you opt for a medical commode, choose a model with backrest and armrests to reduce the risk of falls.

- A bathroom wheelchair can be used both when bathing the patient, and as a portable toilet in the patient's bedroom. It is safer than other mobile toilet alternatives in that it is equipped with a backrest and armrests. You can easily remove the waste collector to empty and clean it.

- Lock all four brakes of the bathroom wheelchair during bathing and when used as a mobile toilet. Otherwise, it will move when you try to transfer the patient to or from it, creating a fall hazard.

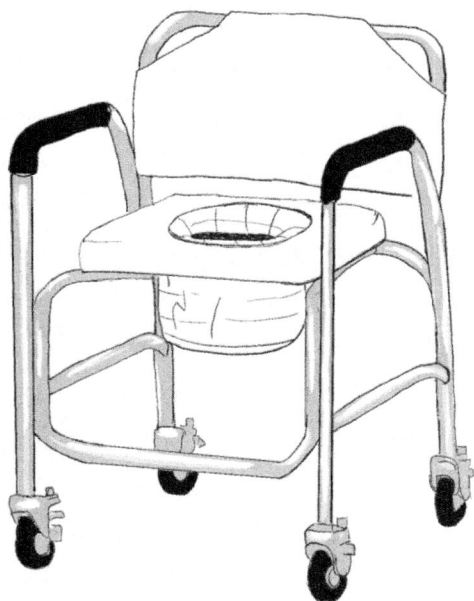

Figure 5.2 Bathroom wheelchair.
Use as a portable toilet or when bathing the patient.

Grab Bars

- Install grab bars at strategic locations in the bathroom so the patient can hold on to them for stability. Grab bars help the patient feel more secure, and therefore more cooperative, when sitting on and getting up from the toilet, and during bath times.

- In the early stage of dementia, the patient can use the bathroom more confidently, while relying on grab bars to help maintain their balance.

- In the middle stage of dementia, you may have the patient hold on to a grab bar while you lower or pull up their pants or otherwise adjust their clothes. Bear in mind, however, that the patient may let go of the grab bar at any time. Stay vigilant and keep an eye on the patient's grip at all times.

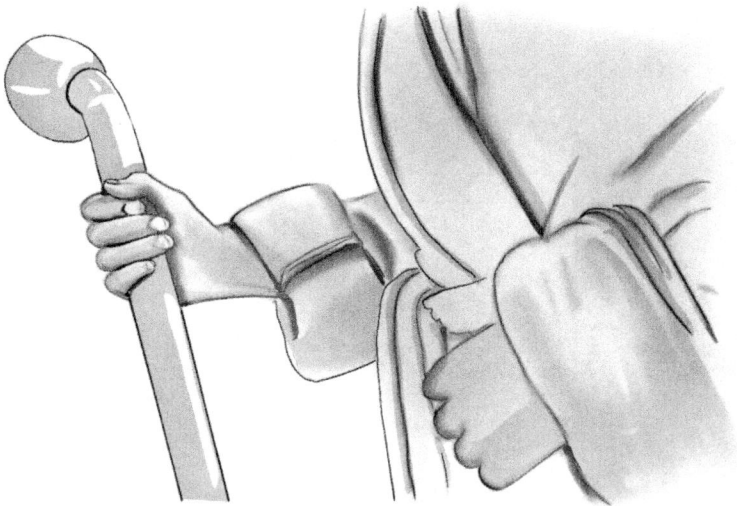

Figure 5.3 Vertical grab bar.
Install grab bars at strategic locations in the bathroom.

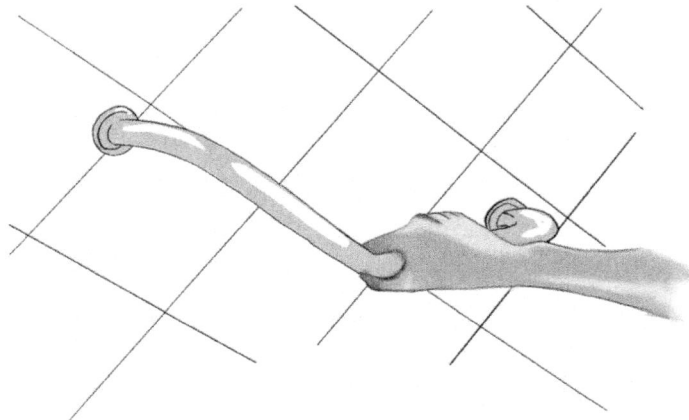

Figure 5.4 Horizontal grab bar.
Have the patient hold on to a grab bar to free up your hands.

Showers and Bathtubs

With dementia, stepping into and out of bathtubs and shower basins quickly becomes impractical. Moreover, a smooth bathtub or shower basin presents an added risk of slips and falls.

- Affix adhesive non-slip stickers to the bathroom floor, bathtubs, and shower basins to reduce the risk of slips.

- Consider installing a walk-in shower designed for the elderly or the disabled. Keep in mind that eventually you'll need room for a wheelchair and a caregiver in addition to the patient.

- A more practical solution would be a bathing room similar to what you'd find at a gym. This would allow for easy wheelchair access and maneuverability by the caregiver who has to walk around the patient to bathe them properly.

- A hand-held showerhead can make the process of bathing easier for both the patient and their caregiver. With a hand-held showerhead, the caregiver can manage the washing more easily, and the patient will not get annoyed or agitated by the noise and the splashing of a fixed showerhead.

Bathing Chair

Before long, standing in the shower will become impractical, and the patient will need to be seated during bathing times.

- Install a bath seat or shower chair in the bathroom for the patient to sit in during bathing. The chair should have a wide base for stability, and a backrest and armrests to prevent falls.

- Choose a chair with a color that stands out against the bathroom floor and walls so the patient can see the chair easily and feel more secure when trying to sit down.

- Bolt the chair to the floor or otherwise fix it in place so it doesn't move. A chair that slips makes it difficult to help the patient into and out of the chair, creating a fall hazard.

Bathroom Wheelchair

Soon, the most practical way to bathe the patient will be to use a bathroom wheelchair.

- You can undress and prepare the patient in a convenient staging area while they are seated in the bathroom wheelchair, then roll the wheelchair into the bathroom.

Faucets and Water Temperature

Adjusting water temperature will grow more difficult over time. Even if the patient is able to wash and bathe on their own, they may need help to prevent scalds.

To help the patient remain independent longer, install faucets that have familiar designs and are easy to use.

- Choose a faucet with separate hot and cold controls, as patients typically find it easier to adjust water temperature with separate controls.

- If you have a choice, opt for a double-lever design with longer levers. The simple push/pull action of the levers makes them easier to operate, especially for patients with arthritis.

- Faucet designs with knob or crosshead controls are harder to use, as the required grasp-and-rotate operation can be difficult and error-prone for patients with dementia.

- More modern designs, such as single-lever combination faucets and electronic faucets with automatic water shutoff, are less familiar than dual-control designs, making it harder for patients to learn and remember how to use them.

- Older bathroom setups with two separate faucets for cold and hot water (rather than two separate controls on a single faucet) are not suitable for patients with dementia, as separate faucets with separate streams of cold and hot water increase the risks of scalding.

Other Bathroom Safety Measures

- Adjust the water heater setting so the hot water is not so hot as to scald the patient.

- Equip the bathroom with adequate lighting.

- Separate the bathroom exhaust fan from the light switch. The noise of the fan may add to the patient's anxiety, or may trigger hallucinations.

- Install a mirror in the bathroom, at a height suitable for the patient to do their grooming. However, keep in mind that the mirror may startle the patient if they are unable to recognize their own image. If so, either remove the mirror or cover it up with some paper or cloth.

- Make sure that the patient cannot lock themselves inside the bathroom. If the latch or lock cannot be opened from the outside, it is best to remove it altogether.

KITCHEN, APPLIANCES, AND TOOLS

My mother put an electric kettle on a gas stove. By the time I realized what had happened, the kettle was on fire and the plastic had melted onto the stove. For her part, Mom was in the living room, oblivious to the smell and smoke coming from the kitchen.

The kitchen is one of the most visited areas of a home. It is also one of the most hazardous areas for a patient who is slowly forgetting how to use it. This is especially true during the early stage of dementia, when the patient is still mobile, believes they are healthy, and hasn't had an accident just yet. Therefore, kitchen safety is one of the first things that must be addressed after a diagnosis of dementia.

Securing the Stove

Both electric and gas stoves present potential dangers. However, gas stoves have the added risk of gas leaks that must be taken very seriously.

- Shut the main gas valve to the stove any time it is not in use. This is to prevent the patient from turning on the stove during the night or when they are alone.

- Stoves that must be lit with matches or a lighter present a higher risk of gas leaks since the patient may turn on the gas and then forget to light it.

- Equip the kitchen with both a smoke detector and a carbon monoxide (CO) detector. Test the devices monthly, and replace their batteries at least once every year.

- Install a fire extinguisher in the kitchen, in an easily accessible location. Inspect the fire extinguisher monthly and have it recharged once a year, or as recommended by its manufacturer.

- Train all members of the household, including any part-time caregiving aides, in the correct use of the fire extinguisher.

Securing Appliances and Kitchen Tools

- Unplug all electrical appliances, and put them away.

- Consider installing a separate power line to supply electrical outlets in the kitchen so you can switch off power to the kitchen at night and when the kitchen is not in use.

- Keep hazardous kitchen tools, including knives, cleavers, and scissors in a safe place and out of reach of the patient. If possible, keep them under lock and key.

Dementia-Friendly Kitchen

- Install transparent doors on cabinets. Place utensils and materials that the patient uses frequently in cabinets with transparent doors so the patient can easily find them.

- Put signs with names or pictures on the drawers and cabinet doors to indicate what's inside. Put a picture of spoons and forks on a drawer containing utensils, or write "Spoons and Forks" on a sticker and affix it to the drawer.

- Choose contrasting colors for drawer and cabinet handles so they are easy to distinguish against the background color of the drawers and the cabinets.

- If you have a choice, opt for kitchen cabinets with sliding doors, or equip existing doors with springs so they close automatically. Cabinet doors that are left open are dangerous and can cause accidents.

Hazardous Materials and Tools

- Keep liquid detergents and basic home cleaners out of reach, and in a safe and locked place. Some of these substances are poisonous. It is not uncommon for patients to ingest some of these supplies and end up in an emergency room.

- Keep hammers, nails, and any carpentry, electrical, mechanical, gardening, and other hand tools and power tools in a safe and locked place. Store away hunting and fishing tools, guns and ammunition, and other weapons.

- Watch out for the patient trying to do cleaning or repair work around the house. Besides the obvious dangers of falling off of a ladder or getting electrocuted, there is the possibility that the patient may take apart plumbing or appliances in an attempt to repair them, then be unable to put them back together.

Mom used to cook lunch early and insist that I eat something before heading out to work. One time the food tasted strange. It had an unusual smell, too. I went sniffing around the kitchen, and found the culprit next to the stove. She had fried the potatoes in dishwashing liquid instead of oil.

Lighting and Color

Dark or dimly lit hallways present special hazards. Shadows and uneven lighting can be confusing and frightening to a patient whose ability to process visual information is on the decline. These problems are more acute in the middle of the night, when the patient is half awake and on their way to the bathroom.

- Make sure each room in the house is evenly lit, and lighting is consistent from room to room. Eliminate light and dark spots, glare, shadows, and dark corners.

- Provide adequate lighting for hallways, especially those leading to the bathroom and the kitchen. Keep the lights on through the night. To save energy, you can install electronic motion sensors to turn on the lights when someone walks nearby.

- Keep the bathroom light on after dark and throughout the night. If the exhaust fan and the light share the same switch, you may have to disconnect the fan so its noise does not add to the patient's stress and anxiety.

- Use diffuse lighting and indirect lighting to reduce glare and to spread light more evenly around the room, reducing shadows.

- Put a nightlight in the patient's bedroom so they can see around their room and find their way to the bathroom at night. Choose a nightlight that does not cast shadows around the room.

- Provide extra lighting during waking hours when the patient is engaged in activities, such as making crafts or grooming. Boost lighting near dressers, in closets, and by the bathroom mirror.

- Make it easy for the patient to control the lights. Choose a light switch with a color that stands out against the wall. Install the light switch at a height that is in the field of view of the patient. Clearly mark the on and off positions of the light switch.

Use Color to Enhance Visibility

Make it easier for the patient to find important objects and places around the house. Use color to help objects stand out so the patient can notice them more easily, and find their way around.

- Mark the pathway to the bathroom with luminous color tape.

- Paint the doors of all the important rooms around the house, including the bathroom, the kitchen, and the bedroom. Use colors that help the doors stand out against the adjacent walls.

- Put a picture of a toilet on the bathroom door, or attach a sign with the word "Toilet" written on it. Make sure the picture or the sign stands out against the background color of the door and is within the patient's field of view.

- Choose door handles with contrasting colors so the patient can more easily see and use them. For easier access, equip doors with easy-to-use lever handles, rather than round doorknobs.

- Choose the patient's furniture and accessories in contrasting colors. A brightly colored side table next to the patient's bed is easier to see and use, and white slippers on a dark carpet are easier to find.

Use Color to Camouflage

Use similar colors to make it harder for the patient to see things you don't want them to see. Camouflage doors and door handles to places you don't want the patient to access, such as a staircase or a basement.

- Camouflage doors by painting them the same color as the adjacent walls, or by hanging a curtain in front of them. Choose a curtain with the same color as the adjacent walls.

- Paint door handles the same color as the rest of the door so they blend in together. Choose round doorknobs to make access more difficult.

Safe Bedroom

During the early and middle stages of dementia, bedroom safety is primarily a nighttime challenge. That's when the patient is more susceptible to confusion and disorientation, and can wander off while their caregiver is asleep. Starting in the middle stage and into the late stage, as the patient grows less mobile, the challenge is increasingly one of safety during procedures such as patient transfers to and from bed.

Early Considerations

- If you live in a two-story home, move the patient's bedroom downstairs.

- Make necessary modifications to make the bedroom wheelchair accessible. Consider the eventuality when you'll need to put a hospital bed in the bedroom.

- Make sure that the patient cannot lock themselves inside their bedroom. If the lock cannot be opened from the outside, remove it altogether.

Furnishing for Comfort and Safety

- Put a picture or a sign on the bedroom door to help the patient identify the room. Similarly, put identifying signage on closets and dresser drawers to indicate what's inside.

- Furnish the patient's bedroom with items of contrasting colors to make it easier for the patient to find and use them.

- If the patient has difficulty recognizing themselves in the mirror, remove mirrors from their bedroom or cover them.

- Equip the room with lights that do not shine directly on the patient's face when they are lying down, so you do not disturb the patient if you need to access the room while they are in bed.

Night Safety

- Install safety features to alert you if the patient leaves their room, especially during the night. You can use motion detectors, baby monitors, or similar devices.

- Put a medical commode or a bathroom wheelchair in the patient's bedroom to reduce the need to walk to the bathroom in the middle of the night. If you use a bathroom wheelchair, make sure its four wheels are locked when it is to be used as a mobile toilet.

- Put a nightlight in the patient's bedroom so they can see around their room and find their way to the medical commode or the bathroom at night. Choose a nightlight that does not cast shadows around the room.

Invest in a Hospital Bed

During the middle and late stages of dementia progression, as the patient grows increasingly bedridden and their care needs grow more complex, a hospital bed can be invaluable for comfort and safety of both the patient and their caregiver.

- Raise the back of the bed to a nearly vertical position when you serve food or liquids to the patient to reduce the risks of food or liquids entering their windpipe.

- Raise the back of the bed when the patient has breathing difficulties. Raising the patient's head and chest to an angle of about 30 degrees will help them breathe easier.

- Adjust the height of the bed when you need to transfer the patient to or from bed. Raising the bed to a comfortable level helps you better manage the weight of the patient, thereby reducing the risks of injury to you and the patient.

- Adjust the height of the bed to a comfortable level when bathing or massaging the patient to minimize strain on your back.

- Hospital beds that are equipped with electric motors make the job of raising or lowering the bed and adjusting the back much easier. Other hospital beds allow these adjustments to be made manually, using a handle.

HOME ALONE

The other day, my mother tried to make coffee using jam instead of coffee. She has forgotten even the simplest tasks around the house but doesn't seem to realize it. I worry that someday she might try to cook with bleach, or worse. We've put away everything that could be hazardous. Someone always follows her wherever she goes. Still, I can't shake the feeling that something can go wrong at any moment.

There comes a time when leaving the patient alone for any length of time is risking tragedy. Misuse of kitchen stove or other appliances, getting locked in the bathroom, falling down the stairs, or using hazardous materials such as bleach to cook with are among the perennial dangers of living with dementia. Even if the patient is able to perform certain tasks on their own, there is always the possibility that today will be the day they'll make a mistake with irreparable consequences.

While the patient is still active and can move around on their own, it's important to help them stay independent as much as possible, for as long as possible. In the meantime, one must always keep a watchful eye for safety.

- Safeguard the patient's independence as much as possible. Let them do things on their own, and offer gentle help and guidance if they get stuck or make a mistake.

- Never leave the patient alone. Shadow them wherever they go and keep a watchful eye for potential hazards.

Planning for Emergencies

If you live alone with the patient, or if you'll be alone with them for some time, have a plan for emergencies. Be prepared for emergencies involving the patient, such as a fall, and emergencies that involve your incapacitation. If something were to happen to you, the patient may not recognize that they need to get help, or may not remember how to do it.

- Give a spare key to your home to a neighbor or a family member who lives nearby. Remove keys from entrance locks so they can be opened from the outside.

- Ask a family member or friend to check up on you on specific time intervals, via phone or text, so they are alerted in a reasonable amount of time if you are incapacitated.

- Make sure that the people checking up on you understand the importance of these calls, and know exactly what to do if you do not answer your phone.

- Review your emergency plan regularly, say once every three months, and update it as necessary. Notify all those involved in the plan of any changes.

- Do an emergency drill at least once every six months to identify problems and fix any shortcomings. Make sure that all those involved in the plan, especially the person who is the first contact point for emergencies, participate in these drills.

- Decide on a specific phone number for emergencies. Save this number in your phone for automatic dialing. Carry your phone with you at all times, and keep it within easy reach, even when you go to bed.

- List all emergency numbers on a card, including ambulance, nearest hospital, fire department, utility services, and police. Place it near the phone or post it on the fridge for easy reference.

- Keep the patient's medical records handy for emergency situations.

6 | DAILY AND WEEKLY PLANNING

The cornerstone of an effective care plan is a consistent daily and weekly schedule. Consistent routines and schedules are a source of comfort for the patient and peace of mind for the caregiver. They provide easy and meaningful answers to questions like "What to do now?" They bring a sense of control, help keep things stable and predictable, and reduce the likelihood that something unexpected will go wrong.

As the patient grows more vulnerable over time, it becomes ever more critical to keep track of their nutrition and hydration, rest and relaxation, health, pain, and comfort. You'll find that things will increasingly need balancing on a knife's edge, and routines are the tools that make this precarious dance possible. Routines also give you the opportunity to make small corrections along the way, and weave tidbits of practical wisdom into the fabric of your daily life. With proper routines in place, you won't have to stay constantly on edge, wondering if you have forgotten something important. You can instead focus on monitoring for subtle changes, and catch looming issues before they develop into full-blown crises.

CREATING MEANINGFUL ROUTINES

Mom would make appointments with friends and then not show up. She blamed them for missed meetings, and we believed her, never suspecting that it is she who forgets. Eventually, many of her friends stopped seeing her.

A daily and weekly plan should account for all the events of the day, as much as possible. Include every regular or predictable detail, such as doctors' appointments, walks in the park, reminiscing with photo albums, visiting friends and family, as well as daily hygiene and the proper timing of meds, meals, and snacks.

Creating a Plan

- Develop a daily routine early in the course of dementia progression, and as soon as possible. It is during this time that the patient is still able to adapt to a schedule relatively easily.

- If possible, involve the patient in the planning process so you incorporate more of what they like into their daily schedule.

- Make a list of people and places that the patient enjoys visiting, as well as tasks and activities that interest the patient the most. Try to include them in the patient's daily and weekly schedule.

- Include easy and relaxing activities that you can do together, like walking in the park, gardening, listening to music, dancing, painting, or reading simple stories together.

- Plan activities around the patient's physical and mental abilities, and in accordance with their stage of dementia progression.

Keep It Stable, Yet Flexible

- Schedule activities based on regular and predictable routines. Keep bedtime and wakeup times consistent. Schedule meals, meds, and activities at set times, every day.

- Keep the daily schedule flexible and evolving to reflect the patient's changing condition during the day, and their evolving abilities over time.

- Schedule more challenging tasks, such as walking or bathing, early in the day or at times when the patient has more energy and tends to be more cooperative.

- Allocate more time for meals, getting dressed, and bathing to avoid the stress that results from rushing things.

- Take a break when the patient seems tired, distracted, or moody. If the patient does not show interest in a particular activity, start another activity or take a break.

Household Chores and Personal Hygiene

Find ways to engage the patient in simple household chores, such as setting the table, preparing meals or salad, dusting, and folding laundry. It's tempting to exclude the patient from such activities because of their declining abilities. Remember, however, that the patient's mind needs to be challenged to stay sharp, just as their muscles need exercise to stay healthy and strong. More than that, involving the patient in household activities helps them feel included, useful, and a valued member of the family.

Schedule personal hygiene routines, such as brushing teeth, going to the bathroom, bathing, and getting dressed. Treat these tasks as activities proper, rather than daily chores to rush through on the way to other activities. Help the patient feel more independent by allocating enough time to these tasks so they can successfully complete them and enjoy a sense of accomplishment as a result.

I was helping my father get dressed to go out. When he tried to put on his pajama pants, I took the pants from him, telling him that that was not appropriate attire for going out. He looked at me, and said, "Why do you keep trying to show me that I am stupid?"

Other Activities to Include

Bear in mind that the specific activity and how well it's done are not important. What matters is that the activity be meaningful and improves the patient's quality of life so they participate in it and feel happy doing so. Try to include activities of various types, such as:

- Mental activities like solving puzzles, reading, storytelling, recalling memories, browsing photo albums and recalling the time and place of photos and the people in them

- Creative activities, such as music, painting, and embroidery

- Physical activities such as exercise, a walk in the park, and light gardening

- Social activities like shopping and visiting friends and relatives

- Spiritual activities such as visiting a place of worship, a shrine, or a nature reserve.

Consider Adult Daycare

In many communities, there are centers that care for dementia patients and the elderly during the day. These centers offer a variety of programs and group activities organized around participants' abilities.

You'll need to visit these centers to make sure that the services provided match the needs of your loved one and are within your budget. The services provided by these centers are different and may be a combination of:

- Daily commute service from home to the center and back

- Diet plans including meals and snacks

- Group programs such as dance, music, painting, and storytelling

- Attention to participants' personal needs, including bathroom visits, medication, and personal hygiene

- Supervision by experienced staff, including nurse and doctor visits, as needed.

HELPING THE PATIENT TO ENGAGE

She kept dialing random numbers on the phone, then asking the person on the other end of the line if she could speak with her daughter. When they'd invariably say that they didn't know who her daughter was, she'd apologize and hang up. Then she'd dial another number at random.

Boredom is a real problem in dementia and can contribute to many behavioral problems. As the patient grows unable to engage in daily tasks, inactivity begins to fill the day. It is not uncommon for dementia patients to end up spending many hours in front of the TV each day.

Boredom and inactivity dull the senses and drive the patient further into isolation. Meaningful activities and play are essential for keeping the patient "warmed up" and engaged, and are vital for the patient's sense of well-being. Over time, however, the patient will need more help to stay involved and participate.

Choosing Activities

Think about what activities the patient likes or might enjoy, and help them participate in those activities.

- Choose activities according to the patient's evolving abilities. They may still be able to paint, sing, or play a musical instrument. Include such activities in their daily schedule.

- Select activities that they enjoy. Pay attention to their reaction and demeanor for clues as to which activities they like, which they find boring, and which activities are beyond their ability.

- Engage the patient in activities that make them feel useful and a valued member of the family. Ask for their help in setting the dinner table, preparing salad, or folding the laundry.

- Do not force the patient to engage in a particular activity, or reprimand them if they don't want to do it.

Keeping the Patient Engaged

- Show the patient how to do an activity using simple, short sentences. Then stay with them and participate in the activity together.

- The patient may need more help with parts of an activity. For example, when cooking, they may need help in measuring the ingredients. Help them with kindness and patience. Make them feel useful by pretending to need their help.

- Do not criticize or blame the patient if they make mistakes. If they are doing something that they enjoy and there is no risk to anyone, let them continue even if they do it wrong.

- Talk to the patient while you do the activity, even if the patient is just watching. Even one-way conversations can help the patient stay involved and feel that they are participating in the activity.

- Keep it light and playful. Add a little mystery, humor, surprise, and encouragement to enliven the atmosphere and help the patient connect and engage.

FUN AND GAMES TO GAIN TRACTION

Turn daily tasks into stories, and activities into play. Keep them fun, narrate the steps, add a little challenge, offer an attainable goal or reward, and mix in lots of encouragement. Try different activities and approaches to find what works, and then tweak it to get the best results.

Storytelling

Listening to stories helps keep the patient engaged, without putting too much cognitive burden on them. Patients usually enjoy simple stories that end happily. Folk stories are often great for this purpose, especially if you narrate the story with feeling and flesh it out with bits of your own creative ad-lib. Ask the patient for help in ending some of the sentences, and make the activity into an engaging experience for both of you.

- Add a story to most things you do. It can be as simple as talking through the steps as you prepare the patient for a bath, or a full narration of a folk tale as you keep them company. Stories help focus the mind on the activity at hand and ward off anxiety.

Storytelling Game

In this type of storytelling, one person starts a fictitious story. The next person continues the line of thought and adds something to the story. This activity goes round the room with each person adding to the plot, mostly using humor. The funnier the story, the better the experience.

Make the experience accessible to the patient by telling the story slowly and using simple words. Wait patiently when it's the patient's turn to participate. Even when the patient is unable to participate by adding to the story, they nevertheless enjoy the fun atmosphere, especially if the story or the manner in which it is told is funny or amusing. You may find that stories involving sudden and simple punch lines are easier for the patient to enjoy, as the combination of surprise and simplicity is somehow easier to grasp.

Other Games and Activities

When engaging in activities, remember that the goal is for the patient to have fun and enjoy the activity. It doesn't matter if they do it incorrectly or fail to observe the rules of the game.

Playing Catch

- Fill a small bag with beans. Gently toss the bag to each other and try to catch it.

- Cut a hole in a board or cardboard. Paint the board in a bright color, and try to throw a small ball into the hole from a distance of a few feet. Alternatively, you can use a bucket or a basket instead of a cardboard cutout.

Puzzles

- Draw simple geometric shapes with a part missing, and ask the patient to finish the drawing.

- Write a simple sentence or proverb, leaving one or more words out, and ask the patient to fill in the blanks.

- Tear up a page from a newspaper or magazine into large pieces and ask the patient to put the pieces back together using masking tape.

- Help the patient put together a jigsaw puzzle.

- Collect different coins and ask the patient to help you organize and count them.

- Put a number of familiar objects like spoons, forks, and plates in a bag or a pillowcase, then take turns pulling an item from the bag and, without looking, try to identify it.

Other Activities

- Help the patient to color children's coloring books.
- Make a ball from wool yarn with the patient's help.
- Help the patient knit simple things, like a scarf.

THE JOY OF REMINISCING

People with dementia usually enjoy reminiscing about the past. During the early stage of dementia progression, the patient may happily recount past events to family and friends. Over time, the patient will forget parts of the story and will readily fabricate new parts in their place, believing that the patchwork is the true story.

Eventually, the patient will forget the names of objects, people, and places. With deepening speech impairment, the patient loses the ability to recount stories of past events. Nevertheless, they continue to enjoy looking at photo albums and video clips of their past experiences.

It is important to keep in mind that reminiscing and storytelling are social activities. Whether in the form of recounting past events, flipping through photo albums, or watching video clips, reminiscing and storytelling work only if the caregiver stays with the patient and participates in the activity.

Photo Albums

Photo albums are great for helping the patient remember people's names, their relationships with the patient, and the time and place of past events. A daily stroll down memory lane, especially with children, can be quite refreshing, and children in particular can help the patient to stay engaged and participate in the conversation.

- Organize photos by subject, such as birthdays, weddings, anniversaries, and travel. Sort them by the date they were taken.

- As part of the daily schedule, review the photo albums with the patient. Encourage them to recount stories of past events with the help of the photo albums. Bear in mind that the goal is to enjoy this activity, not the accuracy of the story being recounted.

- Ask simple questions to help the conversation along. Do not rush the patient, and do not correct them when they make a mistake. Instead, say something like, "I thought this was John, your son."

Childhood

- How many siblings did you have?
- What were the names of your siblings?
- What was your dad's job?
- What did your house look like?
- What was the name of your primary school?
- What were your grandparents like? Tell me about them.

Adolescence

- What kind of clothes did you use to wear?
- What kinds of music did you like?
- Who was your best friend?
- What was the name of your high school?
- Was your school far away? How did you go to school?
- Who was your favorite teacher? What do you remember about him or her?

Adulthood

- Which university or college did you attend?
- What did you study?
- What degree did you get?
- What kind of work did you do after graduation?
- How old were you when you got married?
- What is your spouse's name?
- How many children do you have? What are their names?

Organize the Patient's Life Story

A lasting and memorable activity is to collect and organize photos chronicling the patient's life. With the patient's help, arrange the photos in chronological order, from birth, childhood, and teenage years, to marriage, having children, career, travels, and so on.

Having organized the photos, you can now turn them into a digital album. Physical photo albums and the photos in them will gradually wear out due to repeated handling during the daily and weekly reminiscing. Digital albums, however, can last forever.

You can turn digital photo albums into video clips that the patient will enjoy watching repeatedly. Make different versions for appropriate audiences: one for the patient, with happy memories of healthy times, and a more complete version, with additional footage chronicling the patient's battle with dementia, for the rest of the family. You can even make a special version to be gifted to close relatives and friends.

- Play the happy version of the video regularly for the patient as part of their daily schedule.

Making the Story Into a Video

Use simple photo- or video-editing software to breathe life into your digital album. Crop and trim photos and video clips, and string them together into a digital video, complete with simple effects such as fade in and fade out, and background music and voiceovers.

Putting together a digital life story takes a lot of time and patience, but it will be a rewarding experience. Since you have collected and sorted all the photos already, you're halfway there.

- Scan any old photos that remain to be digitized.

- Add photos in proper sequence to your favorite software.

- Decide how long your finished video should be. Based on that, determine the number of photos to use and the length of time for each slide.

- If you include video clips, their playback time will be added to the length of the final video.

- With each photo, display relevant information like the date of the photo, the location, and any other information you deem appropriate.

- Use special effects thoughtfully. Add motion, filters, and fade in and out to give some sense of movement to the story. But, remember that the story itself must take center stage.

- Add the patient's favorite music to the audio track of the video.

- At the beginning and the end of the video, add any relevant information, like title of the clip, producer's name, soundtrack credits, and credits for people who helped.

KEEPING A DAILY LOG

The other side of a daily and weekly plan is a daily log that faithfully tracks the events of each day. It is the daily log that enables you to monitor the patient's condition as it evolves over time, and to adjust your care plan to meet challenges as they arise. Without a daily log, even the best-laid plans are soon overwhelmed as it becomes impossible to keep track of events over days, weeks, and months.

The daily log is the basis for the update process that keeps the daily and weekly schedule relevant over time. It enables the tweaking of routines to keep pace with the changing care needs of the patient. This in turn helps to improve the quality of life for the patient and their caregivers in subtle and unexpected ways.

Coordinate Among Caregivers

When multiple caregivers are involved in caring for the patient, communication and coordination is vital in ensuring proper care. Everyone involved must follow the planned schedule and record in the daily log all that they do with, and for, the patient. The daily log enables caregivers to be on the same page and find out, at a glance, all the relevant events that have transpired during each other's shift.

The daily log eliminates the need for back-and-forth questions among caregivers regarding patient care. Remember that early in the course of dementia progression, the patient is aware of their problems and highly sensitive to what others say about them. Any discussion of the patient's activities or care needs in their presence can embarrass them and add to their anxiety.

Use the Daily Log to Solve Problems

The daily log is a record of the patient's dementia progression. It details all the activities and events pertaining to patient care, such as changes in behavior, cognition, ability, diet, and medication. When something goes wrong, as it inevitably does, the daily log often holds clues as to the cause, and the key to solving the problem.

- Track changes to the patient's physical and mental condition. Watch for how their dementia is progressing, and how fast. When did they start having trouble using the TV remote? When did they start to have problems with balance? When was the last time they were aggressive?

- Keep track of when you started the patient on a new medication, and stay vigilant for any side effects of the newly administered drugs.

- Keep track of the amount of water and other fluids consumed. Monitor the patient's diet, including snacks. Make sure that they get proper nutrition and hydration.

- Adjust the patient's food and fluid intake with the changing of the seasons, and make the necessary adjustments to their daily and weekly schedule.

- Record the frequency of bathroom visits, including quality and quantity at each visit. These details are critical in preventing constipation or dehydration.

- Schedule bathroom visits frequently and at specific time intervals, like every hour. Adjust the frequency to manage incontinence. While not ultimately preventable, incontinence can be largely managed by regular visits to the bathroom.

- Record qualitative observations such as the patient's mood, behavior, interest in a particular activity or food, or their need for rest and sleep. Discover what activities they enjoy, and include them in their daily schedule.

Sample Daily Log

Figure 6.1 is a sample daily log. Record the date and day of the week on the first line. File the daily reports by date in a binder or folder. Keep them organized so you can easily thumb through them for clues when problems arise.

Record each activity in the appropriate column, with qualitative statements added as necessary. Add or remove columns to meet the needs of your specific situation. Here are sample activities to record, with examples of entries:

- Time of day: "8:00 AM"

- Fluids served – amount, type, and time: "Half a cup of milk at 8:30 AM"

- Food served – amount, type, and time: "Medium banana" or "Small bowl of oatmeal at 9:00 AM." Record all food items like ice cream, almonds, oatmeal, chicken sandwich, coffee, sweets, yogurt, fruits, as well as medications.

- Activities – type, duration, and time: "Storytelling 20 min, at 10:00 AM." Record all activities, such as walking, painting, storytelling, hand and foot massage, shaving, and so on.

- Bathroom – type, time, quantity and quality when appropriate: "Bathroom visit at 11:00 AM." Note quality, quantity, odor, color, whether complete or semi-complete, hard or soft, and so on. Record all hygiene-related activities, including washing hands and face, brushing teeth and hair, trimming nails, shaving and makeup, and bathing.

- Pads and diapers: If the patient uses incontinence pads or diapers, record the time when the pads or diapers were wet or soiled and needed to be changed. With sufficiently frequent bathroom visits, changing of pads usually only happens as part of scheduled bathroom visits.

- Remarks: Record additional comments as necessary, such as, "Was happy with the day's walk," "Drank a glass of milk with appetite," "Paid attention during storytelling," "Took a 20 minute nap," or "Was angry and aggressive" or "Lethargic, anxious." These descriptions are invaluable in keeping track of the progression of dementia, effectiveness and side effects of medications, and the patient's mental and physical ability over time. In the same column, record their blood pressure and temperature at the beginning and at the end of the day.

At the end of each day or shift, record your qualitative observations about the patient in the space provided. Include whether or not they were cooperative, how long they needed to rest, how was their balance, were they talkative or quiet, or any other issue of relevance that may come to mind.

Sun	Mon	Tue	Wed	Thu	Fri	Sat	Date:	
Time	Fluids	Food	Activity	Bathroom		Pads	Remarks
6:00							
7:00							
...							
21:00							
22:00							
22:00 – 6:00								
Observations:								

Figure 6.1 Daily activity log

Appreciate the Good Times

It pains me to watch him melt away, little by little, and it warms my heart when I see the kindness in his eyes and the vulnerability in his demeanor.

Remember that the time period during which you can engage the patient in activities is very short. Over time, the patient's ability to participate in such activities will decline. Treasure the opportunities now and make the most of this time to make new memories.

- Use a smartphone or other device to record memorable interactions with your loved one. Keep your recording device handy so you don't miss any important event.

- In time, you'll come to treasure these recordings as a kind of oral history, to remember the good times you had together, and reminisce about what once was.

- Eventually, the patient will lose the ability to speak and will become housebound and bedridden. By then, even a single "yes" or "no" from them would be a rare gift.

It is tempting to criticize the patient for their repetitive questions, aggression, depression, or other behavioral issues during the early and middle stages of dementia progression. Without a doubt, these will be stressful times that will involve a lot of hard work and sleepless nights. But, there will come a time when you'll look back and long for the days when your loved one was full of energy, active, and even a little mischievous. Eventually, they will quiet down, recede behind weary eyes and, utterly vulnerable, will depend on you for everything.

All the behavioral issues of my dad, all the aggression, anxiety, wandering, and getting lost, all that is history now. He is bedridden and cannot even express his thirst or hunger anymore. I see him losing his grip on life bit by bit, and I long to hear him yell at me one more time.

7 | BEHAVIOR CHANGES

Behavior and personality change with progressing dementia. People with dementia often behave in ways that are very different from their "old self", and these changes can be hard for family and friends to handle. About 30 to 90 percent of dementia patients experience behavior changes at some point during the course of their illness.

Dealing with behavioral changes and coming to terms with them are some of the most stressful and difficult challenges that patients and their families have to face. Still, behavior changes are manageable. With a little detective work, it is usually possible to identify the underlying causes of a behavior problem and correct or manage the behavior, often without resorting to drugs.

SOLVING BEHAVIORAL PROBLEMS

Since my dad was diagnosed five years ago, he's had many mishaps. Giving money to strangers, accusing neighbors of stealing his car, fighting a passerby for no reason... His anger was a real problem: he broke my mom's rib for not getting him what he wanted right away.

Behavioral changes in dementia are a result of ongoing destruction of neurons in the brain. As the network of neurons continues to unravel, the patient's ability to make sense of, and cope with, the world around them is impaired. The patient feels vulnerable, anxious and helpless, and may develop behavioral issues such as aggression, suspicion, depression, hallucinations, and other problems that affect their behavior in profound ways.

Depending on the type of dementia, behavior changes can appear at the start or later on in the course of dementia progression. In Alzheimer's disease, most behavior changes occur in the middle stage of the disease and decline in frequency and intensity over time. In contrast, in frontotemporal dementia, behavior changes are among the primary symptoms and appear before the onset of memory loss.

Managing Behavioral Issues

Although you cannot prevent behavioral changes from happening, you can decrease their frequency, intensity, and duration with creativity, flexibility, kindness, and patience.

- Maintain predictable routines. Over time, the patient's ability to recognize, articulate, or resolve their needs is progressively impaired. As a result, it falls on the caregiver to anticipate and address all of the patient's needs, all the time. A predictable routine helps to reduce behavioral issues by ensuring that the basic needs of the patient are met.

- Remember that the patient is not being difficult on purpose. The changes in their behavior reflect the changes that are taking place in their brain. Although their perception of the world around them may be far from reality, what they perceive is nevertheless quite real to them.

- Appreciate the anxiety, insecurity, and confusion that the patient is likely experiencing. Reassure them with words and action. Caress their hands, hug them, and say kind words to soothe their anxiety.

- Try to find out what is bothering them. Pay attention to their needs and remove any discomfort or pain. Do not press the patient on to do something despite their discomfort, as that may lead to a catastrophic reaction, such as crying, shouting, hitting themselves, throwing things, and so on.

- How you carry yourself affects the patient's psyche and their behavior. Do not engage with the patient when you're angry or emotional. If you're impatient or stressed out, they too will feel the stress and frustration.

- Forcing the patient in any way, belittling them, and getting angry in response to their aggressiveness will only intensify their behavior, and may even end with you losing control of the situation. When necessary, give the patient some space so both of you have time to calm down.

Go With the Flow, and Redirect

There are times when you have to stand up to the patient's wishes. If they want to do something that is dangerous to themselves or others, you must prevent it with all the tricks and creativity that you can muster. If, on the other hand, what they want to do does not pose a risk to anyone, there's no need to intervene. So, if the patient wants to drive, reach into your bag of tricks; if they want to eat with their hands, let them be.

- If the patient insists on wearing a specific item of clothing or if there is a disagreement on how to set the dinner table, ask yourself whether this is a problem that must be resolved right now. If this is a safe environment and there is no danger to anyone, leave the patient alone and correct the action later.

- The patient's behavior may stem from a specific idea in their mind. If they remove all clothes from their dresser, inspect them, and put them right back, perhaps they are bored and want to be doing something useful. Help them meet this need by engaging them in an activity that makes them feel needed and important.

- When possible, help the patient feel independent in their day-to-day activities and reinforce the idea that they are still a valued member of the family. Behavior problems may stem from a feeling of worthlessness, or a feeling that they are a burden on those around them.

Care-Based Interventions

Often, caregivers look for drugs as a solution to behavioral problems, and the use of prescription psychotropic drugs is common, especially in nursing homes. However, in most cases other than severe aggression or depression, drugs may not be the best option.

- Using drugs to mask behavioral issues does not resolve the underlying problem. If the patient is aggressive or cannot sleep due to pain from an underlying illness such as urinary tract infection, medicating the patient with sedatives does not alleviate their suffering.

- Many drugs have unpleasant side effects, such as lethargy and grogginess, that sap energy and quality of life from the patient. Whenever possible try to lighten the patient's physical and mental load, rather than weighing them down with more.

A better way to resolve behavioral issues is to address their underlying causes. Providing for patient health and comfort is the most effective way to handle behavioral issues and to prevent many problems from occurring in the first place. Such care-based interventions have been shown to reduce or eliminate the need for drugs, while at the same time improving the quality of life for the patient and their caregiver.

IDENTIFY CAUSES OF BEHAVIORAL ISSUES

Many factors affect the onset, duration, and intensity of behavior changes. However, the most common triggers of behavioral problems fall along one of three dimensions:

1. Patient
    a. Basic needs
    b. Health conditions
    c. Drug interactions or side effects
2. Environment
3. Caregiver

Examples

Basic needs	Hunger, thirst, pain, other discomfort
Health conditions	Infection, constipation, skin rash
Drug interactions	Start of a new drug, change in dosage
Environment	Hot, cold, noise, crowds
Caregiver	Communication, interaction, trust

Treat Underlying Causes

- Use the behavior change problem solver later in this chapter to identify the factors surrounding the patient's behavior issues. Mark all items that apply to make sure you're not forgetting anything important that may be contributing to the problem.

- Carefully examine, identify, and eliminate the factors that cause or aggravate the behavior change. Start with the most common factors, including urinary tract infection, constipation, visual or hearing impairment, uncomfortable room temperature, children running about, and noise from the TV or other sources.

- Behavioral changes can ebb and flow. A particular behavior, such as aggression, may decrease for a while, then reappear later, or may be more severe one day and less so the next day. The causes for the reappearance or increased severity may be subtle and involve some detective work to decipher.

- At some point, you may find that an intervention that used to work in the past doesn't work anymore. Stay flexible and look for creative solutions. Consult with other caregivers to find approaches that have worked for them in similar situations.

- Consult a doctor if you are unable to identify the causes of behavior changes. In some cases, pain or other conditions such as urinary tract infection, medication side effects, or drug interactions may trigger or aggravate behavior changes. Sometimes a small change in the patient's medications can eliminate the problem. Your doctor will decide if any change to medication is warranted.

- Do not medicate the patient on your own. Do not use sedatives to calm them down. Any medication that is not prescribed by a doctor may have serious adverse consequences, and may make the behavioral problems worse.

Watch for Sudden Loss of Ability

A sudden loss of speech or other abilities is different from the gradual impairment that accompanies dementia progression, and may be a signal that something other than dementia is at work. A sudden loss of speech, and indeed any abrupt change in the patient's alertness, demeanor, or cooperation, may be due to acute or serious medical conditions, such as a stroke, urinary tract infection, or drug interactions or side effects.

Investigate any sudden loss of speech or other abrupt changes in the patient's condition, and seek medical advice if necessary.

- Has the patient taken any new meds? Check for drug side effects and interactions.

- Has the patient's caregiver changed? Has their room changed?

- Is there an underlying health issue, such as constipation, or urinary tract infection?

When to See a Doctor

Consult with your doctor if:

- There is an unexplained sudden loss of ability
- Severe aggression or depression is present
- Behavioral problems do not improve through interventions
- Drug interactions or side effects are suspected
- Problems have medical root causes, such as pain or infection.

When Visiting a Doctor

Take with you:

- A copy of the behavior change problem solver checklist later in this chapter, properly filled out

- A list of the patient's medications, including any supplements

- The patient's medical records.

This information helps your doctor get a full background of any new behavioral issues, helping them home in on possible causes. It also helps you make sure that you do not forget anything important when consulting with your doctor.

LEARN TO READ THE PATIENT

My mother has completely lost the ability to speak. We can't tell what she wants or how she feels, whether she is hungry, thirsty, stressed, or in pain.

In later stages of dementia, finding out if the patient is in pain or has some other need is possible only through vigilance and careful attention by the caregiver. You'll have to infer what is going on from subtle hints in the patient's demeanor. For example, at the onset of urinary tract infection, the patient may not have a fever, and may not be able to communicate their discomfort during urination. The patient's general demeanor, however, provides clues: closed eyes during the day, tendency to sleep more than usual, and lethargy are indications that something is wrong. A caregiver who is on the lookout for warning signs begins to suspect urinary tract infection right away and springs into action to test for and contain the problem.

Reading the patient involves noticing and interpreting subtle clues. This is not possible if there are too many issues going on at the same time. If the patient is simultaneously hungry, thirsty, has urinary tract infection, and is overwhelmed by all the noise around them, it's impossible to discover and tend to all the issues at once. A more practical approach is to ensure that all of the patient's predictable needs are met at all times, leaving the detective work for new and emerging issues only. Only then can you notice subtle changes in the patient's demeanor, and decipher what is going on behind the scenes.

BEHAVIOR CHANGE PROBLEM SOLVER

My mom had undergone surgery. At night, she was restless and wanted to go home. A nurse making rounds asked me how she was. "I don't know how much longer I can keep her in bed," I said. She examined my mom, and said, "I think she's in pain." I told her that my mom hadn't said anything about pain. She nodded, hooking up my mom's morphine. "They don't always tell you when they're in pain."

When trying to solve a new behavior problem, it helps to go through the usual suspects systematically. The following questionnaire is a roundup of the common factors contributing to behavioral issues. It helps you zero in on the underlying causes. Use it when investigating behavioral problems on your own, consulting with other caregivers on a support forum, or seeing your doctor.

Patient Data

When asking a question on a support forum, provide enough information about your particular situation to help others give you relevant advice.

CAUTION: Do not share personal information online.

Patient Info

- Sex: Male / Female
- Age

Type of Dementia

- Alzheimer's disease
- Vascular dementia
- Lewy body dementia
- Frontotemporal dementia
- Mixed dementia (specify the types present)

Progression Stage

- Early stage
- Middle stage
- Late stage

Behavior Problems

- What new behavior problem are you concerned about?
- What other behavior problems were already present?

Select All that Apply

- Boredom
- Aggression
- Stubbornness, uncooperative
- Suspicion
- Illusion
- Insomnia
- Fear
- Anxiety
- Restlessness

- Repetition
- Hoarding
- Depression
- Crying / laughing
- Wandering
- Confusion
- Urinary incontinence
- Fecal incontinence
- Balance problems
- Other

Interventions Attempted

- What interventions have you tried so far to manage the new behavior problem?

- What was the result of each action or intervention tried so far?

Environmental Issues

The environment is typically the most fluid and frequently changing area of the patient's life. So, when investigating a new behavioral problem and rounding up the usual suspects, the environment should be the first on the list.

Is the Patient Overwhelmed?

- Is the patient's environment noisy?
- Are there strangers or other visitors present? (no, a few, many)
- Is the room lighting adequate? (too bright, too dark, okay)
- How is the room temperature? (cold, hot, comfortable)

Is the Patient Bored?

- Are the patient's days organized around routines?

- Does the patient's daily schedule include enough activities?

- Does the patient get eight hours of sleep? More? Less?

Has There Been a Change?

- In caregivers?

- In the patient's room or residence?

- In the patient's medication? (new meds, change in dosage)

Are the Amenities Accessible?

- Does the patient have easy access to the bathroom?

- Are there stairs or other fall hazards in the patient's residence?

- Are there safety grab bars installed everywhere they are needed?

Clinical Observations

The factors relating to the patient's physical health are the most critical and should be examined carefully. Remember that the patient may not be able to express their pain or discomfort. Likewise, they may not exhibit common symptoms of infections, such as a fever.

Pain / Fever

- Does the patient have pain? (mild, severe)

- Does the patient have fever? (low, high)

Eating / Drinking

- Is the patient hungry?
- Is the patient thirsty?
- How is the patient's appetite?
- Has the patient gained or lost weight recently?
- Does the patient have trouble swallowing?
- Do the patient's dentures fit properly?

Urine

- How frequently does the patient urinate?
- What is the color of the urine? (dark indicates dehydration)
- Is there blood in the urine? (dark or brown urine)

Constipation / Diarrhea

- Is the patient constipated?
- Does the patient have diarrhea?

Infection / Other Conditions

- Gum
- Teeth
- Urinary tract
- Lung, pneumonia
- Bed sores
- Other

Underlying Diseases and Conditions

- Hearing problems
- Vision problems
- Arthritis
- Gastric acid reflux
- Diabetes
- High blood pressure
- Cardiac problems
- Vascular disease
- Prostate issues
- Other

Caregiver Interaction

Personal interactions have the potential to soothe and relax, or annoy and aggravate. Evaluate your interactions from the point of view of the patient. How would they rate your bedside manner?

How Does the Caregiver Interact With the Patient?

- Talks down to the patient or uses baby talk
- Uses logic to reason with the patient
- Uses force
- Is rude
- Raises voice
- Threatens
- Strikes the patient

How Is the Caregiver's History With the Patient?

- Good
- Bad (acrimony and conflict)

Relationship of the Caregiver to the Patient

- Spouse
- Son
- Daughter
- Other

BEHAVIOR PROBLEM SOLVER CHECKLIST

Each time you navigate a new behavioral issue, especially one that requires detailed analysis, keep a record of your investigation in the patient's dementia folder, next to the daily log for that day. Use a consistent format, such as the checklist of Figure 7.1, so you can see at a glance the salient features of each analysis. That way, as new problems arise over time, it is easier to thumb through your previous records for clues to help you solve the new problems.

General info	Dementia type	Stage
Sex: male/female Age: Date:	Alzheimer's Vascular Lewy body Frontotemporal Mixed (specify)	Early Middle Late

Behavior issues (existing)

Boredom Aggression Stubbornness Suspicion Illusion Insomnia	Fear Anxiety Restlessness Repetition Hoarding Depression	Crying/laughing Wandering Confusion Urinary incontinence Fecal incontinence Balance problems

Other:

Behavior issues (new):

Interventions attempted and results:

Environment	Changes	Amenities
Noise Visitors Lighting Temperature	Caregiver Room/residence Medication	Bathroom accessible Stairs, fall hazards Safety grab bars

Figure 7.1 Behavior problem solver checklist

Daily schedule		
Days organized around routines Schedule includes adequate activities 8 hours of sleep		

Eating/drinking	Fever/pain	Infection
Hungry Thirsty Appetite Weight gain/loss Swallowing issues Dentures fit	Fever: low/high Pain: mild/severe	Tooth Gum Urinary tract Lung, pneumonia Other:

Bathroom visits	Underlying diseases & conditions	
Frequency Urine color Blood in urine Constipation Diarrhea	Hearing problems Vision problems Arthritis Diabetes Acid reflux	High blood pressure Cardiac problems Vascular disease Prostate issues Other:

Caregiver history	Interaction	Relationship
Good Bad (conflict)	Talks down Uses logic Rude Raises voice Uses force Strikes patient	Spouse Son Daughter Other

Figure 7.1 (continued)

8 | COMMON BEHAVIOR PROBLEMS

Dementia is usually thought of as a disorder of memory and cognition. In practice, however, it is the associated behavioral complications that bring patients and caregivers to their knees. Although behavioral challenges may appear mysterious or irrational at first, they are manageable. If you know how they come about and what they represent, you can better understand how your loved one feels and why. With that knowledge, you are better able to help them cope.

AGGRESSION

I knew something was wrong with me when I started to get into trouble at work. At first, it was arguments over trivial things, but then it escalated. Eventually, I got into a fistfight with another employee, and was fired. I felt relieved. Now I could stay home and watch TV all day. Eventually, I was diagnosed with FTD.

Anger and frustration are common in dementia. As cognitive decline takes its toll, the patient grows less able to tolerate the challenges of daily life or mold the environment to their needs. The situation is made worse by the fact that impulse control is one of the early casualties in some forms of dementia, such as frontotemporal dementia (FTD). With the loss of this critical function, a patient who never had a tendency toward aggression in the past can exhibit surprising levels of rage and aggression seemingly blowing up out of nowhere.

- Do not take it personally. Anger and aggression are caused by the patient's dementia and are not a reflection of their feelings toward you.

- Stay vigilant. Aggression is dangerous and can cause physical and emotional harm to the caregiver or bystanders. Stay alert for its danger signs and never get complacent about them.

- Most patients do better at certain times of the day. When possible, plan their more demanding activities, such as bathing, walking, or exercise, during those hours.

Causes of Aggression

Recently, my dad has become aggressive for no apparent reason. There's been no change in his routine, living environment, caregiver, medication, sleep, or diet.

Aggression can occur for a variety of reasons, including physical discomfort, environmental factors, or communication problems. As with other behavioral problems, one often has to look beyond the obvious to find the reasons for aggression. When a patient is unable to express their pain or discomfort, even a simple headache can go untreated for hours. Look for:

- Physical discomfort such as pain, fever, urinary tract infection, colds, constipation, fatigue, sleep deprivation, sundowning, and insomnia.

- Environmental factors such as a loud TV, children running around, crowds and family gatherings (especially if they include people the patient does not know), high or low ambient temperature, or unsuitable lighting.

- Communication problems such as repeated and complex questions by the caregiver, rushed interaction, or caregiver distress and fatigue. Reduce or eliminate noise, crowds, and other distractions prior to attempting to communicate.

- Drug interactions and side effects, caused by a new medication (including prescription and over-the-counter meds), change in dosage, or mistakes in administering the drugs.

How to Deal With Aggression

I was in the other room checking my email when my mom walked in angry and hit me. I smiled and said, "It's okay Mommy, give all the sweets and candies that you have for me!" At that moment her face lit up and her demeanor changed, and she started caressing my face. It turns out she was upset that I was spending too much time away from her.

- Look for clues right before the onset of aggressive episodes to identify and eliminate the causes of aggression.

- Don't ask the patient why they are angry. Instead, try to find the feelings behind their anger.

- Speak positively to reassure the patient. You can say, "I understand it's difficult for you," or "I understand how hard it is."

- Comfort the patient by maintaining a relaxed demeanor. Speak in a soft and reassuring tone. Remember that even subtle expressions of anxiety and tension in your demeanor may increase the patient's anxiety and agitation.

- Engage with the patient with a confidence that communicates that you trust them and are not afraid of them. Take a deep breath and loosen up before you reach out to the patient.

- Abandon the activity that caused the aggression and do something else. Distract the patient with easy and relaxing activities.

- Lower the risk to yourself and the patient. Keep a safe distance to reduce the chances of getting shoved, hit, or something thrown at you.

- Do not use force. Restraining the patient only adds to their anger and may cause the situation to get out of control.

Have a Plan

Rage and aggression may blow up out of nowhere and at any time. Learn to read the signs in the patient's face and demeanor. Always monitor for physical discomfort, environmental factors, communication issues, and drug-related problems. Have a plan for your safety and that of the patient in case of rage.

- Hide dangerous objects such as kitchen knives, scissors, hammers and other tools. Bear in mind that any object can be thrown and any liquid can be splashed or sprayed.

- If you are living alone with the patient, stay in close contact with family and close friends so they can come to your aid if necessary.

- Have an escape plan for emergencies. Know which exits to use and when. Place emergency supplies such as shoes, a change of clothes, cash, and phone numbers in strategic locations, where you can get to them quickly on your way out. Be prepared to stay out a night or two until you figure out what to do next.

Practice Kindness and Patience

My father was abusive to my sister and me all his life. Now that he has dementia, he still tries to hurt us as we care for him. For a while he had calmed down some, but since last week he's back to the same aggressive person he was at the early stage of his dementia. We try to be kind, but kindness always seems to have the opposite effect on him.

Dementia is often accompanied by a loss of inhibitions. For a person who had been reserved in the past, that may mean singing, dancing, arguing, cursing, or fighting when they become ill. For a person who had been mean or abusive all their life, dementia may make the behavior even worse.

Kindness and patience are the most practical tools in the caregiver's toolbox, even if a patient doesn't make it easy to feel compassion for them. Remember that the patient cannot learn, and scolding or reprimanding them will not improve their behavior. Worse, the toxic physiological and psychological effects of conflict linger long after the episode, setting up the patient and caregiver for more conflict down the line. This reduces the quality of life for everyone involved in incalculable ways.

When to See a Doctor

Seek help if care-based interventions are not successful, or if the aggressive behavior is severe, recurring, lengthy, or if there are risks of harm to the caregiver, patient, or others.

ANXIETY

It is difficult to grasp the depth of anxiety that a person feels as their struggle with dementia unfolds. Forgetfulness, disorientation, and confusion signal the unknown closing in a bit more each day. Uncertainty and vulnerability permeate their existence. Insecurity is a constant companion.

There isn't much a patient can do on their own to soothe their anxiety. What little they can do, they do endlessly. They wring their hands constantly, walk about aimlessly, and engage in compulsive and other self-soothing behaviors.

Recognize Signs of Anxiety

Anxiety is an unpleasant feeling. Stay on the lookout for signs of anxiety so you can take action to soothe a loved one in need of reassurance. Look for:

- Restlessness and walking about aimlessly

- Obsessive-compulsive behaviors such as washing hands a set number of times, or counting the number of steps up and down the stairs

- Self-soothing behaviors such as fiddling with buttons, pulling at threads, folding and creasing a single sheet of tissue paper indefinitely, or wringing their hands until they are raw

- Tension and teeth grinding. The latter occurs in 4 percent of patients with dementia and can eventually lead to broken teeth.

Anxiety Triggers

I used to wash and prep my wife in the morning and help her with her breakfast before heading out to work. One day I had to leave early and couldn't stay for breakfast. That was a difficult day for my wife. She was agitated the whole time I was gone: wouldn't eat, kept going from room to room, repeatedly grabbing the phone and holding it to her ear, then putting it down again. It was only in the evening after I got home and helped her with her dinner that she calmed down and was able to fall asleep.

Any seemingly minor event or a small change in the patient's routine can trigger anxiety. Some of the more common triggers include:

- Fear, fatigue, and hopelessness, and the struggle to understand the environment that is increasingly unfamiliar to them

- Incorrect perception of environmental stimuli, such as street and neighborhood noise, the sound of wind, or lightning

- Psychological stressors, such as death of a loved one, acrimony and conflict, or financial and family problems

- Changes in living conditions, including home, room, caregiver, or transfer to a nursing home, travel, and hospitalization

- Medication issues such as a new medication, changes in timing and dosage, and drug interactions and side effects

- Other health problems such as infections, colds, migraines, skin rash, and joint pain.

How to Deal With Anxiety

Mom is restless. She walks around aimlessly, keeps checking the closet, and is constantly eating something. She hangs the laundry and then goes back in two minutes to see if it has dried already.

Keep a close eye on the demeanor of the patient for any sign of discomfort or anxiety. Try to find the root causes of anxiety and eliminate them. Failure to remove the causes of anxiety can make it worse and may lead to restlessness, anger, and aggression.

- Pay attention to environmental stressors and try to eliminate them. Turn down the TV or radio, ask children to play somewhere else, or move the patient to a quiet place.

- Make sure the patient does not have any pain or discomfort. Watch for full bladder, constipation, infection, skin rash, hunger, thirst, feeling hot or cold, and so on.

- Be relaxed and reassuring. Even subtle signs of agitation in your demeanor will amplify the patient's anxiety. Be their rock, calm and stable, so they can feel safe with you.

- Stay with the patient and comfort them with soothing words. Say things like: "You're safe here," "I'm sorry you feel anxious," or "I'll stay with you until you feel better."

- Soothe with a gentle touch. Kneel in front of the patient's chair so you are at their level, and extend your hands palms up, as if inviting them to put their hands in yours. Then gently pat and massage their hands.

- Take care to not surprise the patient. Approach in a way that they see you coming, and remain constantly in their field of view. Move gently, introduce yourself, and state your relationship. Make eye contact and smile. Avoid sudden or unexpected movements.

- Avoid anxiety-provoking behaviors. Do not restrain the patient, and do not force them to do anything. Never use harsh or demeaning words.

Distract and Redirect

- Distract the patient with relaxing and comforting activities and help them take their mind off of their anxiety.

- Interrupt obsessive-compulsive behavior, such as repeated hand washing, by handing the patient something soft, like a towel, to hold for you. You must appear to genuinely need their help, rather than just trying to get them to stop the compulsive behavior.

- Redirect harmful self-soothing behavior, such as pulling on threads or wringing their hands until they are raw, by handing the patient a small ball to hold and squeeze. Choose a ball that is soft and pliable yet sturdy so it does not open at the seams as a result of the patient's compulsive exploration.

When to See a Doctor

Talk to your doctor if care-based interventions are not successful, or if anxiety lasts for days or worsens. Do not give the patient sedatives or other drugs without a prescription from their doctor. Improper medication can cause more harm than good.

REPETITION

In one of her notebooks, she had discovered a prayer she had written some time ago, the sum of all the hopes and dreams she had had for her children, and she was now reading it. I could hear in her voice how hard she tried to concentrate, each time she started again from the top. She'd start sharp, enunciating each word, and within a sentence or two, she'd be droning on again, mindlessly speeding through the words on the page. Then she'd catch herself, go back to the beginning and start over, each time trying harder to stay focused. Eventually she gave up. "I can't remember what I'm reading," she said with a sigh, clearly exhausted. Then she put away the prayer, stashed it away in her notebook in the middle of so many other notes and reminders she had written to herself over the years. And then she stashed away the notebook.

Repetition is common during the early stage, and sometimes the middle stage, of dementia progression. Patients may repeat daily tasks such as shaving, may collect items obsessively, ask the same question repeatedly, or tell a story over and over again. They may read the first few lines of a story again and again, never getting past the first paragraph, because they keep losing track of what they've just read.

Repetition is primarily a result of short-term memory impairment. The patient does not remember that they told the story or asked the same question moments ago. Other issues such as anxiety and confusion are often contributing factors. In asking repeated questions, the patient may be trying to express a concern, ask for help, or soothe feelings of anxiety, insecurity, and helplessness. Repeated questions may be an attempt to gain reassurance from others, especially their caregiver.

She kept asking if the windows were closed, the door locked, or the stove was off. Sometimes we'd kid her about it. We didn't know any better.

During this phase, the patient becomes attached to their caregiver and shadows them everywhere they go, in what is sometimes called the "Velcro effect." This may be due to feelings of insecurity and anxiety that accompany the profound sense of vulnerability that comes with dementia.

Reassure to Ease Anxiety

- You'll need to be extra patient during this phase. Remember that the patient genuinely does not remember that they asked the same question moments ago.

- Answer questions with simple, short sentences. Stay courteous, even if it is the same question, and the same answer, from moments ago.

- Do not try to convince the patient that you have already answered their question. Even if they understand what you are saying, they will forget it a moment later. Keep in mind that even when reading a simple story, they forget the beginning of a sentence before reaching its end.

- Do not criticize the patient. Blaming the patient, putting them down, and reminding them of their mistakes serves no purpose other than to embarrass the patient, or make them angry.

- Deal with the patient's worries, anxiety, and confusion. Keep calm and stay attentive. Speak in a gentle and reassuring tone. Hold their hands and respond with empathy. Reassure the patient with your calm demeanor to help ease their anxiety.

- Manage the behavior by finding what triggers it. Does the repetition occur in a particular setting, in the presence of a particular person, or at a specific time of the day? Maybe the patient is trying to bring a problem to your attention.

Use Memory Aids

- If the patient's abilities permit it, help them write down the information they need, like the daily schedule and doctors' appointments, in a small pocketbook, mobile phone, or tablet, and refer to it when needed.

- Install a whiteboard in the kitchen or in the patient's bedroom. At the end of each day, erase the board completely and write the next day's schedule for their easy reference.

- At the top of the whiteboard write the day of the week and the date. Specify the day's schedule in simple and easy-to-read format. Note all important activities such as a walk in the park, doctor's appointment, shopping, visiting relatives, and so on.

- Put a calendar with large print and a digital clock in the patient's bedroom. Every night, cross out that day on the calendar using a marker with bold color.

HOARDING

I set out to do my dad a favor by clearing out his room of all the junk and clutter he had collected. I went about the business with my usual gusto, piling the junk outside his room and wondering how anyone could live in such a mess. I'll never forget the look on his face as he watched from the hallway, his hair uneven from the haircut he had given himself earlier that day. When I had finished, I patted myself on the back, proud of the job I had done so quickly, never bothering to ask if he wanted my help, why he had collected all that stuff in the first place, or what it had meant to him.

Hoarding is most commonly seen in Alzheimer's disease, frontotemporal dementia, and Lewy body dementia. Around 23 percent of dementia patients develop hoarding behavior, typically in the early and middle stages of their illness.

Patients hoard all kinds of stuff. They collect, organize, fold and package them, put them away in nooks and crannies, and then spend many busy hours searching in various drawers, cabinets, and wardrobes to rediscover and unpack the items, only to repackage and store them again.

Hoarding typically occurs in tandem with obsessive-compulsive behavior, overeating, and pilfering. What all these behaviors have in common is an underlying sense of anxiety, impairment in impulse control, and memory loss. The patient is trying to get a grip on a life that is increasingly out of their control, with a mind that is no longer able to hold on.

Hoarding is also seen in some older individuals who do not have dementia. Hoarding in older individuals may be a precursor to dementia and a warning sign.

How to Handle Hoarding

Although hoarding can be challenging for the caregiver, it does not help to get angry or scold the patient. Patience, creativity, and humor are better ways of handling all kinds of behavioral problems, and hoarding is no exception.

- Find out what drives the hoarding behavior and try to remove the cause. Is the patient worried that their stuff may get lost or stolen? When they spread, repackage, and store items, are they trying to reassure themselves that they can find the items again? Are they bored from inactivity and a lack of meaningful involvement with the daily household affairs?

- What do they collect and where do they store them? Are the collected items perishable? Are they valuable? By knowing the types of items that the patient likes to collect and where they stash them, you can better decide your next steps.

- Reduce the number of drawers and wardrobes that the patient uses. Label drawers to clearly show what's inside. You can write "socks," "underwear," etc. on sticky notes, then attach the notes to drawers. Or, you can affix pictures to drawers, indicating their contents.

- Make life easy for the patient. Use a large plastic basket for the collected items so the patient can easily find them in one place and pack them again when finished.

- If a particular type of hoarding does not pose a hazard, let it be. But, if the hoarding creates risks, such as food that spoils or clutter that presents a fall hazard, find ways to remove the risk.

- Avoid removing or discarding hoarded items as this may add to the patient's anxiety. Find other ways to remove any risks. For example, if hoarded food has spoiled, replace it with fresh food.

- The patient may agree to donate some of the items to charity. Take this opportunity to quickly remove those items from view. If the patient finds them again, they'll likely hoard them again.

- When going shopping, plan ahead to avoid situations where the patient can re-purchase items they have just discarded. If they come across the same items, they will likely buy them again.

- Do not try to persuade the patient to give up hoarding. They cannot follow your reasoning. Even if you could convince them, they would forget it a few moments later.

- Try to channel their energy to more productive activities like helping to set the dinner table, making salad, and folding laundry.

DEPRESSION

Depression is one of the most common behavioral changes in dementia. It occurs mostly during the early stage, when the patient is more or less aware of their problems. They know that they can no longer remember the names of many of their colleagues and friends. They realize that they are slowly losing their memory and other abilities. They used to be the rock of the family, but now, they worry that they're becoming their family's biggest burden.

Symptoms of Depression

Depression is a disorder that must be dealt with and treated. Symptoms of depression vary, and their severity is not the same in all cases. Common symptoms of depression include:

- Persistent pessimism

- Feeling guilty, worthless, helpless

- Agitation and restlessness

- Loss of interest in activities that used to bring joy

- Feeling tired and lacking energy

- Unexplained aches and pains

- Inability to concentrate or remember details

- Difficulty with everyday decisions

- Changes in appetite resulting in weight gain or loss

- Having suicidal thoughts or attempting suicide.

Helping the Patient Cope

Caring for a loved one who is suffering from depression requires a great deal of energy and patience. It is important to not lose sight of the fact that depression is a symptom of dementia and that the patient is not being lazy. They cannot "snap out of it," and you cannot lift the fog of depression by force. Because the patient's judgment is impaired, you cannot reason with them, either. Instead, use the following tips to help them cope:

- Organize their day around routines. Routines help carry the patient forward through the day and keep them connected to the life that is going on around them.

- Keep routines predictable and regular. Schedule meals and medication times, bedtime and wakeup times, exercise and walks in the park at the same time every day.

- Help the patient engage with life through relaxing and enjoyable activities like walking in the park, gardening, listening to music, dancing, and hand and foot massages. Take them to places they enjoy and have them spend time with people they like.

- Schedule challenging tasks, such as walking or bathing, for when the patient has more energy and is more cooperative, usually early in the day.

- Create a relaxing and inviting atmosphere at home. Cook the meals that they like, and find ways to involve them in simple household chores. Remind them, with kind and appreciative words, that you value them and appreciate their help.

- Be gentle and speak in a soft tone to reassure the patient. If you are anxious or stressed out, your demeanor will drive the patient away, leading to further withdrawal and isolation.

- Acknowledge their depression and give them hope that they will recover soon. Assure them that you will never leave them. Say things like: "I love you," "You're important to me," "I'll never leave you," and "I listen to you, but I cannot possibly fathom the depths of your suffering."

- Do not minimize their pain and do not blame them for their depression. Avoid impractical and discouraging advice. Never say: "Stop whining and complaining," "You are really useless," "If you don't like how you feel, change it," or "Get up and do something."

When to See a Doctor

Consult a doctor if depression is severe and does not resolve through care-based interventions.

APATHY

> *I don't really care for anything or anybody anymore. I love my wife and my children, but somehow, I can't get myself to show them affection anymore. I don't know what's going on with me. Sometimes I get angry and yell at my wife for no reason. Sometimes I get restless and pace and curse at everyone for hours. But at other times, I feel drained of life. I just want to stay in bed until I die.*

Apathy is one of the earlier signs of mild cognitive impairment, which may be a precursor to dementia. Apathy usually appears during the first stage of dementia progression and is often mistaken by family and friends as a byproduct of retirement or old age. In dementia, apathy is the result of the destruction of brain cells in the frontal lobe, the center for judgment and planning. This is one of the first areas of the brain impacted in frontotemporal dementia (FTD) and consequently, symptoms of apathy tend to appear earlier in FTD than in Alzheimer's disease.

Apathy has a profound effect on the quality of life of the patient and their family. As apathy sets in, the patient grows indifferent to things that they used to find moving or enjoyable in the past. They lose interest in family affairs, do not participate in social activities, and do not start any activity on their own. They must be prodded by their caregiver constantly and reminded to do things or stay engaged. Eventually they will lose all connection to the emotional, social, and meaningful aspects of life.

Apathy makes patients socially isolated and may be a precursor to depression. Patients who live with their spouses are less susceptible to apathy than those who live with someone other than a spouse.

Find Creative Ways to Engage

Treat the patient with kindness and empathy. Show them that they are still an important part of the family. Engage with them however you can:

- Involve the patient in activities that they enjoy and are still able to do. Entice them by making the activity fun. Ask their close friends to take them to the park, to the countryside, or other places they used to enjoy in the past.

- Stay flexible and change the activity if necessary. If the patient loses interest halfway through a puzzle, start another activity, like playing cards. Don't worry about the rules of the game or keeping score. Keep it fun and light.

Combine Problems Into Joint Solutions

Dad has FTD. He used to walk a lot, but now he sits in his chair and sleeps all the time. He has gained weight. All he wants is ice cream. Yesterday, I held his hand and we walked around the living room a little bit. He suddenly got agitated and said, "I'm tired. We walked too much."

Combine activities in ways that motivate and moderate each other. Use ice cream to motivate a walk in the park, and a walk in the park to buy time and moderate the demand for ice cream.

- Do not argue. If the patient complains that they haven't had any ice cream, showing them empty wrappers won't help. It is futile to try to reason with the patient. Instead, go with the flow and redirect.

- If the patient wants ice cream, tell them that you'll go and buy ice cream together, then take them to the park instead. Tell them the ice cream shop is on the other side of the park. Use the walk to get some exercise and to buy some time.

- After the walk, have some ice cream and comment about how good it feels to have some ice cream after a walk in the park.

- Help the patient slow down and savor the moment. Make a game of nibbling at the ice cream instead of scarfing it down.

LOSS OF EMPATHY

> *When my dad was diagnosed with a brain tumor and had to operate, my mom didn't show any reaction to the news. She didn't seem worried at all and didn't show the slightest curiosity as to what had happened. When he'd go to see the doctor, she wouldn't go with him. "I don't have time," she'd say, or "This is not that important anyway. We'll see what happens next week."*

Most dementia patients will eventually experience impairment in their ability to feel empathy. The timing and severity of this loss varies among patients and across different types of dementia.

In Alzheimer's disease, problems with empathy appear after memory impairment, and usually after the patient has been diagnosed with dementia. The patient may continue to experience and show empathy through the early stage, and sometimes into the middle stage, of dementia progression. Eventually, however, they will start to show a lack of empathy in their behavior and demeanor.

In contrast, patients with frontotemporal dementia (FTD) typically exhibit a loss of empathy at the early stage of dementia progression. This early onset is due to the loss of gray matter in the region of the brain responsible for social functioning. It usually happens before any noticeable impairment in memory, and often before dementia is suspected. In such cases, loss of empathy may be incorrectly diagnosed as a psychiatric disorder and be treated as such.

In FTD, the loss of empathy is especially painful for the family. The patient insists that they love their spouse and their children, yet do not show any reaction in situations that call for an emotional response. The news of a daughter's engagement, the death of a close friend, or the sight of a grandchild falling down the stairs does not stir any noticeable emotion in the patient.

Because the loss of empathy is due to underlying damage to the brain, any efforts to awaken a sense of empathy in the patient will be in vain. Eventually, the patient will care only about their own needs, and without regard to the needs of anyone else around them. When they'll want something, they'll want it right away, and any delay or resistance on the part of the caregiver will quickly be met with shouting, cursing, and aggression.

Adapting to the New Reality

- Loss of empathy means that the patient cannot process that you are unable to meet their demands right away. Do not try to reason with them or explain that you cannot do something.

- Do not answer the patient with a "No." Instead, respond with a "Yes," and redirect. Say something like: "Yes, dear, we do not have any bananas, but we will buy some when we go to the park this afternoon."

- Do not blame the patient for their insensitivity. Remember that their lack of empathy is due to the ongoing damage in their brain and is out of their control.

- Do not subject the patient to drugs and supplements in the hopes of reawakening empathy. Accept that vast numbers of neurons in their brain have died and continue to die every day, and no amount of nutritional supplements or drugs can make up for that loss.

- The patient cannot change. The sooner you come to terms with that reality, the easier it is for you and the rest of the family to adapt to the new normal. Acceptance is the first step to making peace with the new reality.

INAPPROPRIATE SEXUAL BEHAVIOR

Inappropriate sexual behavior is relatively common in dementia. It occurs in about 7 to 25 percent of patients and is more prevalent in nursing homes. In men, the behavior tends to be more explicit and physical, while in women it's often verbal and less explicit.

Inappropriate sexual behavior may occur anywhere: at home in front of family and friends or outside in plain view of strangers. Patients with access to the Internet may become obsessive in visiting porn sites or purchasing magazines and other forms of pornography. They become easy targets for financial or other forms of abuse and scams.

Improper sexual behavior is a consequence of damage to the frontal lobes of the brain, and the resulting impairment in judgment and impulse control. Consequently, it tends to occur earlier in frontotemporal dementia (FTD) than in Alzheimer's disease. FTD is associated with a slew of other impairments in executive function as a result of damage to the frontal lobes, making it difficult to correct patient behavior through explanations and reasoning.

Dementia and Sex

During the course of dementia, the patient's ability to engage in sexual activity evolves in ways that parallel the decline in other abilities. Just as the patient gradually loses track of the steps involved in brushing their teeth, grooming, or bathing, sooner or later they begin to forget the steps involved in intimate relationships and may need more help to stay sexually active.

Over time, the patient becomes oblivious to the needs of their partner, may try to engage in unusual sex acts, or may even commit sexual violence. Forgetting that they had been intimate with their partner moments ago, the patient may want to do it again, and may get angry when they are refused. As with other behavioral problems, distracting the patient is usually more effective, and potentially safer, than an outright "No!"

Sexual Behavior in Nursing Homes

Most of the research into inappropriate sexual behavior has focused on nursing homes. Their findings and solutions, however, are equally applicable to patients living at home.

- Drug-based interventions are more prevalent at nursing homes because of their ease of use and a shortage of trained staff. However, care-based interventions are often more effective at helping with behavioral problems, including sexual issues.

- In nursing homes, it is recommended that patients reside in single rooms. The ladies' and men's wards should be separate and on different floors, and served by female and male staff respectively. TV programs and print materials should be controlled for content that may be sexually arousing.

- Tell the patient when a particular behavior is inappropriate. If a male patient enters the room of a female patient, gently direct him to his own room, and say something like: "Gentlemen should not enter ladies' rooms."

- Educational interventions, including explanations, are less likely to work with dementia patients, however. Memory problems make it difficult for dementia patients to learn and remember, while impaired reasoning and impulse control make it difficult for patients to follow your logic or redirect their behavior.

Managing Sexual Behavior

Reduce inappropriate sexual behavior by anticipating it and redirecting the patient. In both these areas you have a significant advantage: you can see farther into the future than the patient and can hold on to a thought or a strategy longer than they can.

- Distracting the patient remains one of the most effective tools in helping with behavior issues. This is especially true for sexual behaviors, as a hard and fast refusal, and the resulting feelings of rejection, can trigger a more angry or violent response.

- The patient may approach strangers in a store or at a park, and act in an inappropriate manner, like hugging them. To prevent this, always place yourself between the patient and strangers so you can intervene and redirect as necessary.

- Watch for urinary tract infection and constipation. These conditions and their resulting discomfort may attract the patient's attention to their genitals, creating the impression that the behavior is sexually motivated.

- If the patient tends to reach down their pants or take their clothes off at inappropriate times, make it harder for them to do so by having them wear closed-front or one-piece clothes.

Dealing With the Stigma

Inappropriate sexual behavior can be especially embarrassing for the caregiver or other members of the family due to the stigma associated with it.

- Remember that inappropriate sexual behavior is a consequence of dementia, and not the result of some moral failing or character flaw on the part of the patient, or a shortcoming on your part as a spouse or partner.

- Educate yourself about changes in sexual behavior and the evolving sexual needs of the patient. A better understanding of the changes helps to reduce the stress of dealing with them. It can also help prolong intimacy between partners, sometimes well into the course of dementia progression.

- Discuss the patient's sexual behavior changes with their doctor, and get practical advice on how to deal with them. People often hesitate to discuss sexual issues with their doctor. As a result, problems with sexual behavior tend to go unresolved.

CONFUSION

I was helping my mother flip through photo albums. I pointed to myself in one of the photos and asked, "Who is this?" She responded, "It's my beautiful daughter." I asked, "Then, who am I?" She stared at me deeply, not knowing how to answer.

Confusion is a consequence of short-term memory loss and the resulting impairment of cognitive processes that depend on short-term memory. When one cannot hold on to a thought or a step in a process, it is easy to get lost as to what to do next.

Memory loss and confusion appear at different times across the various types of dementia. Confusion tends to occur earlier in Alzheimer's disease, where short-term memory is one of the first areas affected, while in frontotemporal dementia and Parkinson's disease dementia, memory loss and confusion tend to occur in later stages of dementia progression.

At the early stages of memory impairment, the patient may have difficulty remembering events from recent past, have difficulty in day-to-day decision-making, or have a hard time following and participating in conversations. Over time, memory impairment and confusion progressively worsen. The patient may no longer recognize family members, remember their names, or understand their relationships. They may forget how to use a fork or a pencil, and what purpose they serve.

Reduce Cognitive Load

With advancing dementia, as brain function is increasingly impaired, it becomes easier for outside stimuli to overwhelm the brain's information processing capacity, leading to confusion. Anything that adds to the cognitive load on the patient can quickly add to their confusion.

- Changes in living environment, relocation to a new home or a new room, transfer to a nursing home, or hospitalization are major sources of confusion. Environmental stimuli from visitors, crowds, radio and TV are among others.

- Changes to daily routines can increase confusion. Reduce cognitive load by maintaining predictable daily routines for everything, from meal times to walks in the park, sleep and wakeup times, and other activities during the day.

- Cold and flu, urinary tract infection, pain, constipation, dehydration, and other health-related issues negatively impact cognition and increase patient confusion. Remember that dementia patients usually have difficulty expressing their pain or discomfort. Treat increased confusion as a warning sign that underlying health issues may be at work.

How to Manage Confusion

I was away for three weeks on business. During that time, my mom and I talked on the phone frequently. But, when I got back, she didn't recognize me. It took half a day for her to warm up to me again. I asked her if she knew who I was, and she said my aunt's name instead.

- It is deeply distressing when a loved one calls you by a wrong name or is unable to remember who you are. Stay calm and do not show your sadness.

- Be mindful of your demeanor. Reassure the patient through your body language and tone of voice. Remember that any anxiety or stress on your part will make the patient stressed and anxious in turn, increasing their confusion.

- Do not try to reason with the patient or try to convince them that they are mistaken. They cannot follow your reasoning and may instead get frustrated or angry.

- To help the patient, you have to inhabit their world to some extent. Put yourself in their imagined time and place and help steer them in the real world.

- Use photo albums and memorabilia to help the patient remember. Photos of weddings, graduations, children, and grandchildren can refresh their memory and help them regain their bearings.

- If you need to correct the patient, express it as a suggestion. For example, you can say: "I think he's your son, John," or "I thought it was a pen."

- Speak in short, simple sentences. Speak slowly to give the patient time to process what you are saying.

Reduce Risks Arising From Confusion

- Be mindful of dangers arising from confusion. The patient may leave home at odd hours wearing inappropriate clothing and get lost. They may go to the kitchen, turn on the stove, and leave. At the store, they may put an item in their pocket and forget to pay for it.

- Equip your home with safety devices, such as smoke detectors and door alarms. Make your home dementia friendly by installing appropriate lighting, eliminating safety hazards, and removing dangerous items such as knives, power tools, and chemicals.

WANDERING

Pretty soon, she didn't recognize her own home. But she recognized her furniture. She kept asking why we had brought her stuff to this house, and kept asking that we take her to her own home.

Wandering is a major concern for caregivers. Sixty percent of patients with dementia will wander at least once during the course of their illness. No matter how vigilant you are, chances are that in a brief moment when the patient is out of your sight, they will wander off. If you notice their absence immediately, you might be able to find them in a nearby alley or street. However, there is a real chance that you will not and will have to mobilize family, friends, and the police to search for the patient. It may take days to find a missing loved one, and the longer it takes, the greater the risk for the patient.

When Is Wandering Most Likely?

Dementia patients may not remember their name, may forget their home address, and may lose their sense of orientation in familiar places. If the patient is constantly asking about where they are, if they are restless, if they want to go "home" when they are, in fact, home, or if they have trouble finding familiar places like the bathroom and the kitchen, then the probability of wandering off and getting lost is significant.

$$\begin{array}{c} Ability\ to \\ Walk \end{array} + \begin{array}{c} Memory \\ Impairment \end{array} = \begin{array}{c} Risk\ of\ Wandering \\ and\ Getting\ Lost \end{array}$$

Wandering is sometimes triggered by a desire to go "home." Keep in mind that "home" might mean the patient's current residence, their childhood home, or some other place that looks and feels familiar. Other triggers include forgetfulness, boredom, and loneliness.

Reducing the Risks

To reduce the chances of wandering, ensure that the patient's needs are being met, their anxiety is under control, and they are in a safe environment. It is, however, essential to plan for their safe return in case they do wander off and get lost.

Meet the Patient's Basic Needs

- Make sure the patient's basic needs are met. Are they thirsty or hungry? Are they comfortable? Are they lonely? Do they need to go to the bathroom?

- Try to schedule their fluid intake so they don't drink anything at least two hours before bedtime. Having to go to the bathroom in the middle of the night can be confusing and may increase the chances of wandering.

- Help the patient deplete their pent-up energy with fun activities. Physical activities are great, but any activity will do, as long as it is done in a safe environment and in your presence.

- Organize daily routines around consistent schedules so the activities and events of the day proceed in a habitual way, reducing the likelihood of the patient wandering off in search of something.

- If the patient feels confused or lonely, stay with them and reassure them. You can say, "We're safe here," or "I will stay with you." Or if they want to go "home," tell them "We'll stay here tonight and rest. We will go home tomorrow."

- If they want to leave the house, do not use force or try to reason with them to change their mind. If you can't distract the patient, get dressed and go out with them.

- Never leave the patient alone in the car or at home. The risk of wandering off in such cases is significantly higher.

Implement Safety Measures at Home

- Keep the patient's room, hallways, corridors, and anywhere else they frequent around the house properly lit at all times.

- Equip their bedroom with indirect night lighting. Keep the hallway and bathroom lights on at night, or equip them with motion detectors so when the patient walks nearby the lights turn on.

- The patient may forget the layout of their home or the location of the bathroom, kitchen, or other rooms. Put picture signs on doors to indicate their use. For example, place a picture of a toilet on the bathroom door.

- Lock doors to the outside and remove the keys. If possible, install locks where they will be out of the patient's line of sight, such as high on the door. Camouflage locks and doorknobs by painting them the same color as the door or by covering them up with a curtain.

- Install a bell or an electronic alarm on doors to the outside so you'll know right away if the patient tries to leave the house.

- Hide the car keys to prevent the patient from getting behind the wheel.

Familiarize Yourself With Your Home's Surroundings

- Survey your home's immediate surroundings methodically. Is there any renovation, excavation, drilling, or roadwork going on in the area? Are there empty trenches, water canals, or bluffs nearby? Is your home near busy streets or highways?

- When searching for the patient, keep in mind that right-handed people have a tendency to turn right and left-handed people tend to turn left when they wander.

- Inform neighbors about the patient's dementia, so if they see the patient confused and stranded nearby, they can help them find their way back home, or if necessary, call you.

Facilitate the Patient's Safe Return

- Prepare business cards with the patient's name, phone number, and address. On the back of the card note relevant conditions, such as dementia, diabetes, and so on. Laminate the cards for durability, and place one card in the patient's pocket and another in their wallet or purse, where they can be found by the police or others trying to help the patient.

- Another option is to make a bracelet or pendant with the essential information engraved on it. The patient may be more inclined to wear a jewelry-type ornament, ensuring that the information is always with them.

- If they carry a mobile phone, store emergency contact information in their phone so the contacts are the first items visible in the phonebook.

- You may also use the GPS feature of the patient's phone, or other electronic tracking device, to track the whereabouts of the patient in case they wander off and get lost.

My wife and I had gone to the movies. When she went to use the restroom in the lobby, I stood guard at the entrance holding her purse, my eyes peeled to make sure I wouldn't miss her when she walked out. Five minutes passed, then 10, and then 15. The bustle of people walking in and out of the ladies room had tapered off, and still there was no sign of my wife. I asked someone passing by if she could look inside to see if my wife was alright. A moment later she came back. "There's no one in there," she said. Panic had begun to take hold of me when she said, "You know, this bathroom has another entrance in the next hallway, right by the exit." Frantic, I ran around the corner toward the exit and found my wife alone in the hallway. She was standing by the other entrance to the ladies room, tears streaming down her face, thinking I had abandoned her.

SUNDOWNING AND NIGHTTIME ISSUES

Many of the symptoms of dementia tend to get worse late in the day and toward the evening. During the day the patient might be able to go about their life without too much difficulty, while in late afternoon or evening they may experience increased confusion, restlessness, and anxiety. This is known as sundowning because the confusion tends to intensify during the dusk hours.

Sundowning occurs mostly in the middle and late stages of dementia. The compounding loss of brain cells over time makes it harder for the brain to process complex visual stimuli, such as the dimming ambient light and the lengthening shadows at dusk. Destruction of neurons in the brain also disrupts the body's internal clock, which regulates night and day cycles (circadian rhythms) and related physiological processes. The result is a variety of sleep disorders that reach well past dusk and into the night.

Most elderly people do not enjoy a continuous eight hours of sleep and may wake up several times during the night. For those suffering from dementia, these sleep breaks can be accompanied with confusion of time and place, restlessness, and other behavior disorders. For example, the patient may wake up in the middle of the night, get dressed, and leave home, believing that it is time to go to work.

Improve the Living Environment

- Provide adequate lighting in the patient's living environment. Dim light makes it harder to see things, leading to confusion and anxiety.

- At the end of the day before it gets dark outside, draw the curtains and turn on the lights to make it easier for the patient to transition from day to night.

- Ensure a safe sleeping environment. Equip the patient's room for comfort and safety, including comfortable temperature, nightlight, and closed and locked windows.

- Install safety features to alert you if the patient leaves their room. You can use motion detectors, baby monitors, or similar devices.

- Pay attention to nighttime dangers. The patient may leave home in the middle of the night and not be able to find their way back. Or they may go into the kitchen, turn on the stove, and leave.

Refine Daily Routines

- Organize daily routines with a natural progression from morning to noon, through the dusk hours, and into the night. By the time you help the patient to bed, they should be primed and ready for a good night's sleep.

- Schedule adequate physical activity during the day and prevent long naps. Long naps during the day translate to difficulty sleeping at night.

- Keep dinners light, while lunches can be more filling.

- Avoid coffee, tea, soda, sweets, and alcohol in the evening.

- Limit sensory stimuli during nighttime. Watch out for loud TV, noisy children, and lengthy visits from friends and relatives.

Reduce Physical and Mental Distress

- Watch for signs of physical and mental distress. Hunger or thirst, uncomfortable ambient temperature, fever, constipation, itching, and infection can disrupt the patient's sleep.

- Do not resort to force to put the patient to bed. Restraining the patient in any way and using force will make the situation worse and lead to more anxiety and even aggression.

- Speak gently and make the patient feel safe. Say things like: "Everything is fine," or "Don't worry, I will stay with you."

- If the patient suffers from sleep apnea (a sleep disorder in which breathing stops repeatedly during sleep), consult with your doctor.

Nighttime Pajama Problems

Mom wakes up in the middle of the night and roams around with her pants off. Every time I wake up to check on her, I see her wandering without her pants.

Nighttime problems with diapers, pajamas, and other clothing are common. It may be due to incontinence, discomfort, or confusion. Solve nighttime problems step by step.

- Identify the cause of the behavior. Does the patient have a skin rash or allergies? Are there signs of injury to their skin? Are they suffering from urinary tract infection? Do they feel hot at night? Do they need to use the bathroom?

- The patient may need to use the bathroom at night, and have difficulty putting their pants back on afterwards. Bathroom visits will be easier if the patient is wearing a loose-fitting T-shirt and pull-up pants.

- If pull-up pants are impractical because the patient tends to put their hands down their pants, have them wear a one-piece sleepwear, or union suit, with no opening in the front.

- If you're making a one-piece sleepwear yourself, choose a more durable material and sew the seams several times to make them harder to tear. For the opening in the back, use Velcro instead of zippers and buttons so it is comfortable when the patient sleeps on their back.

- If the patient resists wearing one-piece pajamas, buy two sets of similar attire with colors that they like. Put them side by side on the bed and tell them that you bought two sets for both of you. Ask them to choose the one that they like more.

SUSPICION AND DELUSION

A person with dementia may suspect or accuse others of theft, infidelity, or other impropriety. This can make for some awkward situations at family gatherings, where the patient may openly accuse someone in front of others. Unfounded suspicion, and more broadly delusion, can take many forms, including believing that someone is following or spying on them, that family members betray or steal from them, that the words and actions of public figures are directed at them personally, or that the events depicted in books, poems, newspapers, and movies are about them. While such beliefs have no basis in reality, the patient nevertheless believes them to be true. Delusional thinking usually occurs early in the course of dementia progression and may persist for a long time.

Help Others Respond Appropriately

- Make sure everyone understands that the patient's behavior is not malicious and that it is dementia that is at the root of it.

- Give the accused party a heads-up so they are not taken by surprise in the event that the patient openly accuses them in the presence of others.

- Do not take accusations at face value, and do not take offense, respond defensively, or try to fight the accusations.

- Deal with the patient with understanding and compassion. Stay cordial. Be more of a listener than a speaker. Keep in mind that these beliefs are quite real to the patient.

- If the patient has gifted an item and now believes the item has been stolen, ask the recipient not to wear the item in front of the patient, or better yet, return the item.

Dealing With Delusion

- Do not try to convince the patient that they are mistaken. Remember that their judgment is impaired and they are not able to follow your reasoning. Trying to convince them may even lead to aggression.

- Try instead to find the reasons behind the suspicion and, if possible, eliminate them.

- If the patient believes something has been stolen, help them find the missing item or replace it with a new one. If they have gifted an item, ask the recipient to return the item.

- Be mindful of your demeanor. Speak in a calm and reassuring tone. Stay relaxed and help the patient calm down.

- Do not endorse suspicions and do not try to refute them. Instead, try to distract the patient with something else.

- Use relaxing and easy activities, like a walk outside, to divert the patient's attention to something else.

HALLUCINATION

> *She talked nonstop, sometimes through the night. She talked at length with dead relatives, and when they'd offer her some food, she'd politely accept and eat it. The meds her doctor had prescribed couldn't get her to sleep. Eventually, after twenty-four hours, having completely worn herself out, she'd settle down and sleep for a whole day.*

Hallucination is a condition where the patient sees someone or hears their voice in the absence of actual external stimuli. The patient may see a friend's face in the folds of a curtain or think there's a stranger somewhere in their home. They may see a parent who passed away years ago, hold a conversation with a friend who is not there, or even try to serve them something to eat or drink. Although none of this is real, the experience is nevertheless quite real to the patient, and any attempt to convince them otherwise would be futile.

Hallucinations occur in most types of dementia, and visual hallucinations are the most common type. The duration and severity of hallucinations vary across different types of dementia. In Lewy Body Dementia, this condition is usually more severe and lasts longer.

Helping the Patient Cope

- Do not argue with the patient. Trying to convince them that they are mistaken is futile. It may even lead to aggression.

- Remember that the patient is not trying to deceive you. What they experience is quite real to them. Do not scold or accuse them of lying. Instead, express your love, care, and support.

- Stay with the patient and reassure them. Say things like: "Don't worry, I will stay with you and protect you."

- Try to understand what they are hearing, seeing, and thinking. Find out in what situation, time, and place they find themselves. Adjust your reaction accordingly.

- Try easy and relaxing activities to distract the patient and redirect their attention.

Eliminate Environmental Triggers

- Reduce sensory stimuli. Excessive noise, including TV, music, or a running air conditioner, can trigger hallucinations.

- Too much, or too little, stimulation may trigger hallucinations. If the presence of others is creating problems, take the patient to a quieter and more familiar environment, such as their bedroom. If being alone makes them see or hear things, take them to where others are present.

- Due to the effects of sundowning, confusion and hallucination are more likely at dusk. As the sunset approaches, turn on the lights and draw the curtains to eliminate shadows.

- Eliminate strong reflections. Bright light reflecting on shiny surfaces can create problems.

- Looking in the mirror, the patient may not recognize the person looking back at them. Cover mirrors or remove them from the patient's room.

Address Medical Factors

- Tend to failing eyesight or hearing loss, if present. Does the patient need new eyeglasses? Do they suffer from cataracts? Do they need new hearing aids?

- Examine the patient's physical condition. Are they constipated? Do they have a skin rash, fever, pain, or urinary tract infection? Consult with your doctor when necessary.

Is It Really Hallucination?

Dad keeps hearing people calling him from a distance. He answers in a loud voice, but there's nobody there. This usually happens before he goes to sleep at night or shortly after he wakes up in the morning.

Sometimes it is difficult to tell the difference between hallucination and other conditions such as illusion, delusion, or delirium. The problem is compounded by the fact that the patient is often unable to articulate what they are experiencing. As a result, it may take some detective work to determine which condition is present. Proper detection is critical, however, since each symptom is a clue to underlying conditions and a possible warning sign that may need to be addressed right away.

Illusion

It is near sunset. A gentle breeze moves the curtains. Grandpa believes someone is hiding behind the curtains. You turn on the light and pull the curtains aside. He sees that no one is there and accepts that he was mistaken.

In the case of illusion, the patient misperceives or misinterprets external stimuli, such as a sight or a sound, and confuses one thing for another. They may think that patterns on a rug are live insects or a belt is a snake. They may mistake a distant sound for someone calling, and may get dressed and leave home to investigate. However, they can usually be convinced that they are mistaken.

Delusion

Grandpa is convinced that a neighbor is hiding behind the bushes and is spying on him. You take him outside and show him that there's no one hiding there. He accepts that no one is there but still believes the neighbor is spying on him.

Delusion is rooted in an internal belief, rather than external or internal stimuli. The patient does not see or hear things, real or imagined. The belief exists on its own.

Confusion

> *My mother lost her dad when she was in her twenties. Recently, she asks about him often and wants to go visit him. She remembers the names of other deceased relatives and asks about them, one by one, as if they are still alive.*

Dementia patients often ask about deceased relatives as if they are still alive. This may be a result of memory loss (forgetting that a parent has passed on long ago), or a consequence of not being able to differentiate between past memories and the present. Similarly, patients might speak to a person in a photo or think that a person on the TV screen can see them. This may be a result of difficulty distinguishing images from the people they represent.

As with hallucination, do not try to convince the patient that a parent or relative is no longer alive or try to explain that an image cannot hear them. If the behavior does not pose a danger to the patient or others, let it be. But, if the patient starts to get agitated, sad, or anxious, try to distract them as best as you can.

When to See a Doctor

Talk to your doctor if hallucinations are severe and involve multiple senses, persist for a long time, or happen frequently.

Delirium

Grandpa spent the early hours of the evening with family. But a couple of hours later, he has a fever and is lying in bed. He whines and talks incoherently. We don't know what he sees or says; he doesn't know either. He is half awake and half asleep.

Delirium is not a symptom of dementia. Rather, delirium signals a potentially serious medical condition such as infection, kidney or liver problems, or prescription drug interactions or side effects. It is usually accompanied by fever, sweating, changes in heart rate (increase or decrease), and changes in sleep patterns.

Unlike behavioral changes that are caused by dementia, delirium appears abruptly. It is marked by dramatic and rapid changes in the patient's perception, attention, mood, speech, and ability to move or perform tasks. It appears within a few hours to several days of an underlying condition, and generally disappears if the underlying condition is properly treated.

Delirium is easily confused with behavioral issues such as hallucination, especially in patients who are no longer able to express themselves clearly. As a result, caregivers may fail to take action quickly enough, thereby delaying treatment and allowing the underlying condition to get worse.

- Delirium is a symptom of potentially serious medical conditions that need medical attention right away.

- Delirium may not be accompanied by fever all the time. Therefore in all cases of delirium, consult a doctor.

- People with delirium may do things that are quite dangerous, without realizing the danger, or even remembering doing them afterwards. Do not leave the patient alone.

9 | MAKING SENSE OF THE WORLD

The five senses are the bridges that link us to our environment. They continuously receive information from the world around us, and process it into meaningful knowledge, to construct a mental map of the world in which we find ourselves. Our senses help us connect with the world, make sense of what is happening around us, and react to it appropriately.

The natural process of aging takes its toll on sensory organs. However, age-related vision loss, cataracts, and hearing loss can largely be corrected with the help of hearing aids, eyeglasses, and in some cases, surgery. With dementia, however, it is the sensory processing system that begins to be impaired, making it increasingly difficult to make sense of, and respond to, the world.

DEMENTIA AND THE FIVE SENSES

The phone rang and Mom picked up. "Hello... yes..." Then she drifted off. After a minute or two of silence I asked who was on the phone. "I don't know," she said, still holding the phone to her ear. I took the phone, but there was no one on the line. I asked when did they hang up. She said she didn't know.

People suffering from dementia experience impaired sensory function beyond what is a natural consequence of aging. During the course of dementia progression, patients' sensory and cognitive systems are progressively impaired, making it harder for the brain to receive adequate information about the environment, or to correctly process the information it does receive. As a result, patients' relationship with the world around them is greatly affected.

Because these problems are usually irreversible, it falls on the caregiver to assist the patient in making sense of their environment, for example, by describing external stimuli to the patient and by reducing distractions.

Making Sense of Impaired Senses

My husband came down the stairs and asked what I was doing. "Cleaning the basement," I said, as I continued with the work. He stood there for a minute watching me. Then he came closer and complemented me for the job I was doing. He said he was sorry for not being able to help around the house much anymore and asked if I would be willing to come to his home and help his wife with the housework.

A while later, I had cleaned up and was serving him his lunch. He asked about the lady cleaning downstairs. When I said that she had gone home, he got angry, scolding me for letting the poor woman go on an empty stomach.

Do not be surprised by the patient's unexpected reaction or seemingly odd behavior. Remember that their reaction is due to physical impairments in their sensory and cognitive systems.

- They may receive incomplete information due to problems with sensory organs or signal transmission to the brain.

- They may be unable to properly make sense of sensory inputs due to the progressive neuronal damage in the brain.

As a result, the patient's responses may not be what you expect. You cannot eliminate such problems with logical reasoning, reminders, force, or by humiliating the patient. The patient's condition cannot be reversed. It is the responsibility of the caregiver to adapt to the changing circumstances and to help the patient cope.

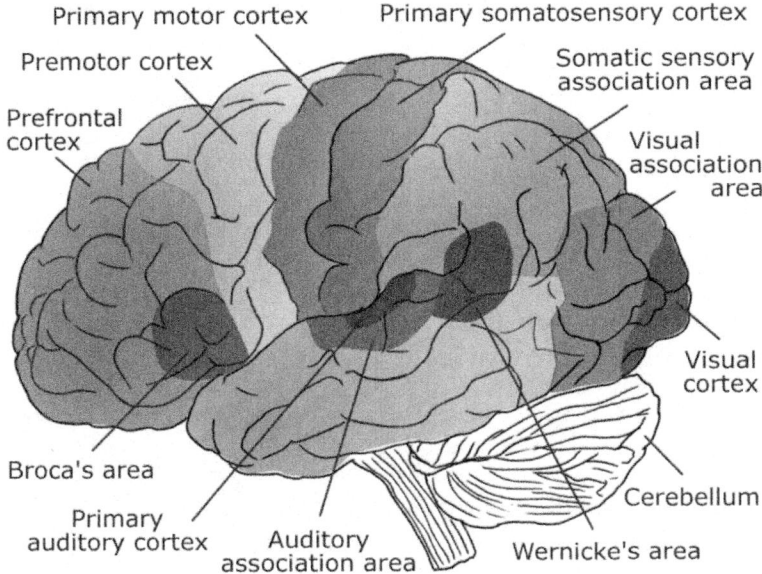

Figure 9.1 Functional areas of the brain

Prefrontal cortex – higher cognitive functions, including judgment, planning, attention, and impulse control.

Primary motor cortex – execution of voluntary movement and muscle control; contains a broad representation of different body parts from toe to mouth.

Secondary motor (premotor) cortex – internal planning of voluntary movements, as opposed to the execution of those voluntary movements.

Broca's area – speech production, including putting thoughts into words, using words and grammar accurately, and monitoring and adjusting the flow of speech.

Primary somatic sensory cortex – sensations from muscles and skin; contains a broad representation of different body parts from toe to mouth.

Somatic sensory association area – perception of touch, weight, texture, temperature, pain, and sense of self-movement and body position.

Visual cortex – vision; receives sensory information from the eyes.

Visual association area – perception of color, distance, size, depth, movement, and identifying objects and faces.

Primary auditory cortex – hearing; receives sensory information from the ears.

Auditory association area – processing information into meaningful units, including sounds, speech, and music.

Wernicke's area – comprehension of written and spoken language

Temporal lobe (other than auditory) – memory, emotional regulation, perception of emotions in facial and auditory stimuli, social cognition.

Cerebellum – coordination of movement, balance, equilibrium, and posture.

Figure 9.1 (continued)

VISION

The sense of sight plays a dominant role in our connection to the outside world. About 80 to 85 percent of our perception and engagement with the world is mediated through vision. With dementia, as cells die and neural pathways are disrupted, visual processing is degraded. The patient will have increasing trouble with visual and spatial relationships, impacting their perception of reality in profound and debilitating ways.

Dementia and Vision

Dementia impairs visual perception in fundamental ways, including by disrupting depth perception, peripheral vision, color, and contrast.

- The patient will have difficulty gauging distances. They may misjudge the height of steps, or have difficulty picking up their cup from a table.

- The visual field narrows and the patient will have difficulty seeing objects and people that are not directly in front of them.

- They will have a hard time deciphering color and contrast. For example, they may not be able to distinguish a white towel from white tiling in the bathroom.

- They may perceive one thing to be something else, like thinking that a coat on a coat hanger is a person standing in the closet, or the patterns on a rug are objects, plants, or insects.

- Face perception may be impaired. The patient may misidentify people, thinking, for example, that their son is their brother.

Simplify the Visual Environment

Make it easier for the patient to see and navigate their living environment. Reduce visual and spatial clutter, and improve lighting and color to help with perception.

- At home, clear the areas that the patient frequents from extra furniture and other obstacles to ease navigation and reduce the risk of falls.

- When walking with the patient, let them know where you're going, in which direction, and any obstacles, like steps or doorjambs, as you encounter them.

- Make sure that the patient's living environment and hallways are well illuminated.

- Choose colors to increase visual contrast. Use contrasting colors for items that the patient uses on a daily basis. Pay special attention to the colors of carpeting, floor tiles, walls, doorknobs, light switches, and bathroom fixtures.

Improving Communication

A consequence of visual impairment is that the patient gradually loses the ability to decipher nonverbal cues during communication. Since an estimated 60 to 90 percent of all communication is nonverbal, this amounts to a substantial impairment in the patient's ability to understand what is going on. As a result, it is up to you to help the patient make sense of their interactions with you and others.

- Approach the patient gently and always with a smile, as though this is the first time you see them today. Communicate a sense of safety and comfort through relaxed and gentle movements.

- The patient may not be able to recognize their visitors' faces. When people visit, announce their names to help the patient know who is present.

- Stay in the patient's direct line of sight so they can see you easily. Impairment in peripheral vision results in a narrowing of field of vision, so if you are not directly in front of the patient, they may not notice your presence.

- Your body language affects the patient more than your words. Avoid gestures that may be perceived as threatening, such as pointing your index finger when talking to them.

- Pay attention to your mood and demeanor when you interact with the patient or are in their vicinity. They can pick up on your stress or agitation from your voice and your demeanor.

HEARING

I don't answer the phone anymore; I can't understand what the other party is saying, nor can I come up with a response in time. I can still write okay, because I can do it slowly and make corrections before sharing it with others.

Over time, dementia affects the auditory and related areas in the brain, resulting in impairments in hearing, speech comprehension, and related functions. Just how much ability the patient retains at any stage can be hard to determine. For example, it is possible that the patient can hear your voice but has difficulty processing it to understand what is being said.

As the auditory areas in the brain are progressively impaired, it becomes increasingly difficult for the brain to break up the continuous stream of auditory information into meaningful units, like individual voices, musical themes, auditory signals such as the ringing of a bell, and words and phrases. As a result, the once-familiar sound environment transforms into a cacophony of sounds grating on the patient's ears. Worse, unlike with sight, the patient has no way of blocking the auditory noise from assaulting their senses, especially in the later stages of dementia progression.

Soften the Auditory Environment

Reduce distractions to lower the cognitive load on the patient. Use sound to soothe rather than overwhelm and confuse the patient.

- Reduce noise from TV, radio, children, and other sources, so the patient can better decipher what is going on around them.

- Play the patient's favorite music. Bear in mind that what they are able to enjoy today may be different from what they used to enjoy in the past.

- Convey emotions through the sound of your voice. Speak in a soothing voice. Whisper words of love and gratitude, even if the patient is unable to understand what you are saying.

Simplify Communication

To help the patient understand, reduce environmental distractions and noise. Adopt a comforting tone, speak slowly, enunciate clearly, and use simple words and constructs.

- The patient will gradually speak in simpler words and concepts. Match your communication style to theirs.

- Use simple words and short sentences. Avoid complex or abstract constructs such as metaphors and sarcasm.

- Stay on one subject at a time. Give the patient time to process one step before moving on to the next. Do not rush through the steps, and do not jump from one subject to another.

- Use proper body language, including hand and face gestures, to facilitate comprehension.

- Pay attention to your tone of voice. Any stress and anxiety in your voice carries through to the patient and drowns out the words and meaning you're trying to get across.

- If the patient cannot understand what you are saying, speaking louder will not make things any better, and may instead make the patient more anxious.

TOUCH

Dementia patients may be unable to properly process some of the sensations associated with touch. They may have difficulty distinguishing between a cold and a hot object or gauge its temperature. However, even in the late stage of dementia, they will enjoy human contact and connection through touch.

Use Touch to Connect

Touch has the power to soothe and improve well-being. It is also an effective way to engage and connect with the patient.

- Before attempting to communicate with the patient, use gentle touch to get their attention. Caress their hands to give their mind a bit of stimulation and a bit of time to warm up.

- Take every opportunity to connect with the patient. Take their hand in yours and gently caress it. Caress their forearms too.

- Hug the patient often and whisper soothing words in their ear. Hold the embrace long enough for the sensation to register.

Use Massage to Soothe

Daily rubdowns and massages are effective in soothing anxiety and improving patients' mood. Over time, as the patient grows less active, massages will become the primary means of providing relief to muscles that must be tired from hours of sitting motionless or lying in bed.

- Use simple massages and rubdowns throughout the day to increase blood flow and soothe the patient's aching limbs.

- Give the patient small massages often during the course of each day. Schedule more thorough massages a few of times a week.

- Massage hands and feet, neck and shoulders, upper and lower back, and arms and legs.

- Use lotions and natural oils to give the patient a full body massage. A good time for this is during bath times.

TASTE

With progressing dementia, the ability to sense saltiness and sweetness tends to be impaired sooner than the ability to sense sourness and bitterness. To make up for this loss of taste, the patient may add more salt to their food, or add more sugar to their tea or coffee. In some cases, one of the first symptoms of dementia is a change in the patient's sense of taste. For example, patients with frontotemporal dementia often develop a sweet tooth.

The Evolving Relationship With Food

- The patient may start finding faults with your cooking. They may like a meal and eat it willingly one day, then criticize you for that same meal on another day. Don't get discouraged, and don't argue with them. Telling them "This is the same meal you enjoyed last time" won't get you anywhere.

- Prepare foods that have both taste and texture. Jam or French fries may be more enticing to the patient than pudding, due to their distinct texture.

- As swallowing problems develop, the patient may forget to swallow the food or medicine already in their mouth. Often a small spoon of ice cream or other food with a completely different taste and texture is enough to get the swallowing process going again.

- Use clever tricks to keep the patient from consuming too much salt or sugar. Remove the saltshaker from the table so it's not within their easy reach or in their line of sight. Serve their tea or coffee with one or two sugar cubes, rather than leaving the sugar bowl in plain view.

That's Not Food!

Dementia patients may put all sorts of things in their mouth, in the same way that toddlers do. They may ingest non-food or poisonous substances, such as paper towels, cigarette butts, and liquid detergents, and end up in the emergency room.

- Do not leave paper towels, cigarettes, pills, and other small objects lying around. Stay vigilant to prevent the patient from ingesting non-food items.

- Keep liquid detergents and basic home cleaners out of reach, and in a safe and locked place. Some of these substances are especially dangerous if ingested.

SMELL

The sense of smell changes significantly over the course of dementia progression. While the patient may still enjoy the smell of newly baked cake and fresh bread, they may have difficulty recognizing some other odors, such as spoiled food or bleach.

When the Safety System No Longer Works

It is hard to appreciate just how much we depend on the sense of smell to keep us out of trouble. When this vital function is impaired, it takes a lot of vigilance to make up for it and ensure safety.

- Discard spoiled foods promptly. The patient may eat spoiled leftover food and get ill.

- Keep disinfectants and cleaning products out of reach. The patient may not be able to smell the pungent odor of bleach, and may drink it.

- Shut the gas supply to the kitchen stove when not in use. The patient may turn on the gas and, unable to smell it, may forget about it and leave the kitchen.

- Watch the patient's hygiene carefully. They may wear clothes that have become soiled due to incontinence; or, unable to sense their own body odor, may refuse to take a bath.

Tapping Into Happy Memories

The olfactory receptors directly project to the amygdala, the area in the brain responsible for processing emotions. This makes the sense of smell closely linked with emotions, and a strong trigger of past memories.

- Apply perfume and other fragrances that the patient likes and used to wear in the past.

- Help the patient enjoy the smell of fresh bread and other triggers of joyful memories.

- Prepare their favorite meals and help them savor the smell, as well as the taste.

- Hug the patient often, and hold the embrace long enough for the patient to take in your scent.

CONNECTING THROUGH THE FIVE SENSES

When cognition is impaired and sensory channels are degraded, connect across multiple sensory modalities to get through.

- Play the patient's favorite music. Dance to the music, even if the patient can only watch. Put on a happy show.

- Read memorable passages from their favorite books. Vary your tone of voice as appropriate, and add facial and hand gestures to enrich the experience.

- Flip through old photo albums and talk about people, places, and shared experiences.

- Prepare their favorite meals.

- Comb, color, and style their hair.

- Massage their hands and feet with scented lotions.

- Take the patient to the backyard or a nearby park in their wheelchair, and spin a few rounds. Then sit together holding hands, and watch birds and flowers, and life, go about the business of living.

10 | COMMUNICATION

With the onset of dementia, as sensory and cognitive systems begin to be impaired, more complex processes that build on those systems are impacted as well. As a result, communication, connection, and understanding are often early casualties of dementia.

- The ability to process sensory information will grow impaired over time, making it harder for the patient to make sense of their environment.

- The patient will have more difficulty operating in the realm of words and concepts, or processing how things relate to each other logically, and across space and time.

When concepts and words are no longer available, communication has to take place through other means, such as touch, feelings, emotion, empathy, quiet moments together, and any other mode of connection that does not rely on abstractions. Without the convenience of words, one is left with no option but to tune in and be present in the moment, to slow down and get quiet, so one can hear what is not being said.

WHEN WORDS FAIL

I had taken my dad to take care of some paperwork. When the clerk asked to "see" his ID, my dad promptly took off his glasses and tried to hand them over instead. Whenever I think about this episode, my heart warms at the thought of my dad's innocence and the genuine way he was trying to comply with the clerk's request. I felt so embarrassed at the time. I wish we had laughed together instead, when he realized his mistake right away.

More and more, the patient will have trouble finding words, and may instead use the wrong words, like saying "pants" when they mean "shoes." The problem here is not necessarily that the patient has forgotten what a shoe is or what the word "shoe" means. Rather, it may be the result of a glitch anywhere in the complex circuitry linking perception to concepts to meaning to intent to motor coordination, or anything else involved in producing speech. Interestingly, the patient usually realizes their mistake right away and can laugh with you if you approach the situation with humor.

Laugh Together

Use humor to reduce tension and anxiety, and foster connection and togetherness. Laugh with the patient, and not at them. Be playful and find ways to laugh together at mishaps of the day.

- If the patient uses the wrong word, like referring to the curtain as "the closet," playfully ask, "The closet?!" Wait for the patient to realize their mistake and then laugh with them.

- If the patient's pants get wet from incontinence, ask playfully, "Wow! Who spilled water on you?" You'll be surprised at how comforting and pleasant things turn out when you approach problems with a little bit of thoughtful humor.

Use a Picture Dictionary

Starting in the middle stage of dementia, the patient will start to have difficulty remembering the names of individuals, objects, places, and foods. Use a picture dictionary to help the patient find the right words and help you understand what they're trying to say.

1. With your phone or a digital camera, take pictures of family members, foods, ingredients, appliances, clothes, body parts such as hands and feet, as well as any other people or objects connected with the patient's daily life.

2. Have the photos printed, and organize them in a photo album. Write the name of the person, object, food, etc. under each photo. Alternatively, you may organize the images in a digital photo album for use on a tablet.

3. Keep the album nearby, and help the patient refer to it as needed.

"I Want to Go Home"

Over time, as it becomes harder to find the right words, the patient will rely increasingly on word substitutions. Sometimes, a word is just meant as a placeholder in a sentence, like saying "Give me my pants" when they want their shoes. At other times, it is the feeling behind the words, rather than their literal meaning, that is intended, for example, "I want to go home."

When the patient says that they want to go home, this is not always due to confusion. Rather, the patient may be expressing a desire for love, peace, comfort, and security that they associate with home. When the patient feels anxious and isolated, when they feel that no one understands them, that everyone is reprimanding them, bossing them around, or asking them to do the impossible, "I want to go home" expresses a need for escape to a familiar shelter, a longing for the warmth and security that they associate with home.

•   Do not try to convince the patient that they are already home. Instead, look for the sentiment behind the words "I want to go home."

- Apply the techniques you'd use to get to the root cause of behavioral problems. Look for unmet needs, environmental issues, and problems with patient-caregiver interactions.

- Are the patient's basic needs being met? Is the patient hungry, thirsty, or in pain? Are they bored? Do they have an infection? Are they constipated, or do they need to go to the bathroom?

- Is the environment comfortable? Is it too warm or too cold, too bright or too dark, too noisy, or crowded?

- Are patient-caregiver interactions thoughtful and comforting? Does the patient feel safe? Do they feel loved, cared for, and accepted? Are they comforted with hugs, caresses, companionship, and words of encouragement?

- Go with the flow and redirect. Say something like, "Okay, we'll go soon," and then distract the patient by doing something pleasant that takes their mind off of wanting to go home.

LOSING TIME AND PLACE

Mom wouldn't eat until everyone had been served, and that meant all her grown children, regardless of where they were in the world. We'd help her box their food and hand it to an imaginary mailman waiting by the door, and the food would be delivered instantly. She had lost all sense of time and place; next door or halfway around the world, dead or alive, were all the same to her. Sometimes, she'd insist on speaking to her children on the phone to make sure they had received the food she had just packed for them. Years later, when she had to be fed one spoonful at a time, we'd tell her that John and Sammy and others wouldn't eat unless she ate, too. And that usually was enough to get her to accept the next bite.

At some point, dementia patients lose all sense of time and place. They may ask about deceased relatives as if they are still alive, or might think it rude to eat or talk in front of a person on the TV screen. In these situations, it is futile, even counterproductive, to try to convince the patient that they are mistaken. Instead, try to inhabit their world. Share in the patient's reality so you can help steer them in the real world.

Go With the Flow, and Redirect

My mother keeps saying that she wants to go to her own home. She says her young kids are home alone. A walk in the park makes her forget for a while, but as soon as we return, she remembers and wants to go home to her kids.

Often, the patient may confuse distant memories with recent past. Old memories of having young children feel new. Distant memories of deceased parents feel fresh, like they are from yesterday. The patient may ask when their father will be home, or may want to go home to be with their young children.

- When the patient asks about a deceased relative, don't tell them that the person passed away a long time ago. The realization may be akin to losing the person all over again.

- Don't try to correct the patient or convince them that they are mistaken. Remember that their memories and feelings are quite real to them.

- To connect with the patient, you have to inhabit their world to some extent. Go with the flow of their thinking and redirect.

- Say something like, "We'll go see the kids after we prepare the salad," or "Your dad will come after breakfast."

- Change the subject, and make the patient focus on something different. Try to keep the patient engaged in doing something meaningful so they can feel helpful and appreciated.

Shield the Patient

My mother has been asking about my cousin, who passed away today. I don't know what to tell her or whether to let her attend the funeral services.

It's often risky to tell the patient about their illness or other bad news such as death of a loved one. This is especially true during the early stage of dementia when the patient is still able to understand the news but is not as emotionally resilient as before. At this stage, words matter greatly, and a thoughtless comment can adversely affect the patient's condition in significant ways.

- In the early stage of dementia, shield the patient from bad news and difficult emotional situations.

- Screen incoming calls from family and friends calling to express their sympathies.

- Tell the patient that the deceased person has gone on a trip, or give some other convincing explanation for their absence.

By the middle or late stage of dementia, the issue is likely moot, as the patient's cognition is largely impaired and apathy has set in. At that point, the patient will no longer show much of a reaction to the news at all.

Don't Overdo Trickery

We conspired to give Mom a nice surprise. We had someone call our home to say that Mom had won the lottery. I picked up the phone and acted all surprised and delighted at the news. Mom bought the story hook, line, and sinker. For days after that, relatives who were in on the story would call to congratulate her on her good fortune. This made her happy for a while.

The ease with which you can trick someone who has dementia is both a blessing and a curse. It can be used in creative ways to get them to go along with what you need to do, without a fight. It also makes the patient susceptible to swindle and abuse by scammers. Before you try to manipulate the patient in any way, remember that even with the best of intentions, it is still manipulation. If the patient gets the feeling that they were scammed, they will not trust you again. Worse, the experience may feed into their suspicion, delusion, and other behavior problems and make them worse.

- Always consider whether the patient would approve of the trick you're about to pull, if they were healthy. Remember that even with the best of intentions, it's not just the end result that matters, but also how you get there.

HOW TO COMMUNICATE

I don't understand some people. Some of our relatives, when they come to visit, don't even try to talk to my mom, or say hello to her, or hold her hands. They act like she's not even there. What's the matter? Why do they even come for a visit? When they meet someone with dementia, do they forget how to behave, too?

It's true that a person with dementia may not remember. But they can still feel. When you're impatient, they know. If you make fun of them, they get upset. When you disrespect them, they feel sad. But when you treat them with dignity, when you treat them with empathy and kindness, they perk up. They look. They pay attention.

Sooner or later, the patient's ability to speak will be impaired. The timing of speech loss varies across different types of dementia and among patients. Patients with Alzheimer's disease may retain the ability to speak into the late stage of the disease, while in some types of frontotemporal dementia speech is an early casualty of the illness.

Understanding the Patient

My mom's speech has become vague and garbled, to the point that I can't understand what she is trying to say anymore. When she says something, I take the easy way out and say okay, then continue with whatever I was doing.

When the patient tries to communicate with you, they are expressing a need that should be addressed. It could be as simple as a need for connection, to have a moment of togetherness, or to feel included in whatever that is going on around them. Or it could be that they are hungry, thirsty, uncomfortable, or in pain.

1. Sit next to the patient. Hold their hand in yours and gently caress it. Give them your undivided attention.

2. Try to find out what they need by asking simple questions requiring yes/no answers. Bear in mind that the patient may answer no when they actually mean yes. Ask things like: Are you thirsty? Do you want some orange juice? Is the room too hot? Do you have pain? Do you need to go to the bathroom?

3. Take your time. Do not rush the patient. Sometimes the process of trying to solve a problem is itself the solution.

Reduce Cognitive Load

My mom speaks very little. Sometimes, if we ask a question several times, she responds with a single word or facial expression.

Over time, it becomes necessary to simplify the patient's environment before attempting to communicate with them. As the patient's cognitive capacity declines, you'll have to reduce their cognitive load, especially during demanding activities such as communication.

• Eliminate distractions when communicating with the patient. Turn off the TV, ask others to keep quiet, or if necessary, leave the room. Alternatively, you can take the patient to a secluded area, like their bedroom.

- Stay in the patient's field of view. Face the patient and get their attention. Use eye contact, and employ hand and facial gestures to make your point. Do not cover your face or mouth when communicating with the patient.

- Be mindful of your demeanor. Stay relaxed and speak in a soft tone. Reassure the patient by staying calm, caring, and attentive.

- Speak in simple, clear, and short sentences. If the patient does not understand, express yourself in another way.

- Ask questions that are easy to process. Instead of "What would you like for lunch?" ask, "Do you want soup or salad for lunch?" or better yet, "Do you want soup?"

Structure Your Interactions

Just as your demeanor and body language are often more important than the actual words being spoken, the way you start and end an interaction is just as critical in helping the patient understand and cope with what is going on.

1. Each time you approach the patient for an interaction, introduce yourself again and declare the reason for the interaction.

2. As you interact with the patient, describe the work you are doing step by step, as you are doing it, in simple short sentences.

3. When you are done, inform the patient before leaving the room.

GOING DEEPER TO CONNECTION

I had just finished with the morning routine of washing and prepping my wife for breakfast. As I parked her wheelchair in front of the fish tank, I spoke to her like I do every day, trying to engage her. I pointed to the colorful fish swimming around in the tank, telling her stories, asking her if she would like to go to faraway places and see exotic fish swimming in the ocean. Trying hard to sound cheerful, I said, "My, dear R., this is our time, our golden years. We're supposed to be together, traveling the world. Why did you get sick?" I didn't worry about the words because I knew she couldn't understand them anymore. And yet, there it was on that day, a tear rolling down her cheek. And I just fell apart.

Communication is not just about transferring facts and ideas from one mind to another. It's about making a connection. Long after the patient loses the ability to speak or understand words, they can still experience connection. Direct touch, gentle sentiments, empathy, and affection operate at more subtle levels than words and concepts. Throughout the course of dementia, and long before words and concepts lose their meaning, communication should extend more and more into the unspoken realm.

Focus your efforts on providing comfort to the patient and to ease the profound anxiety that they are likely experiencing. Hug them at every opportunity and hold the embrace long enough for the sensation to register. Tell them that you love them, and have a heart-to-heart talk, even if the exchange is one-sided. You'll see them react to you with facial expressions, even if they cannot utter a word.

The way you interact with the patient has a profound effect on both of you, including on blood pressure, stress hormones, and neurotransmitters in the brain. The effects of the interaction will remain with the patient, even if they do not remember what happened or why. Simple, seemingly inconsequential events now, impact how the patient responds to unrelated events an hour or more down the line.

- Watch your own physical and mental health. If you are stressed, exhausted, or burnt out, your condition will affect how the patient experiences the interaction. Your emotional state reflects in the patient who can no longer be distracted by words camouflaging your true feelings.

SOOTHING TOUCH

My wife had been on pureed food for some time, when a dear friend came to visit. She looked over our daily schedule, asked about hand, foot, and shoulder massages in our daily routine and then decided to give my wife a full-body massage before giving her a bath. To my surprise and amazement, my wife started eating regular food again. Needless to say, full-body massage is now a mainstay of our weekly schedule.

Dementia invokes a great deal of anxiety, as evidenced by patients' constant wringing of the hands and other self-soothing behaviors. Touch is a powerful soothing mechanism. It is also a path to deeper connection and intimacy. Make touch part of the patient's daily schedule, like diet and hydration, to make sure they receive as much as you think they're getting.

Hug

Hug the patient at every opportunity. Hold them in your arms and whisper your gratitude for what they have meant to you all these years. Express your appreciation for all that they have done in the past. Tell them you love them and hold them dear. You might be surprised at the effect such expressions of affection and gratitude have on both of you.

Caress

Hold the patient's hand in yours and caress it. Gently caress the patient's forehead, eyebrows, temples, and cheeks. Speak softly as you take in the intimacy of the moment. Notice the vulnerability and trust in their eyes. The possibility of connection is still there, if you remember to look for it.

Massage

Regular, gentle, and frequent massages during the day help relax the patient's muscles and prevent their limbs from stiffening up or locking in place. Massage is a helpful substitute for physical activity, especially in later stages of dementia when the patient is no longer able to move on their own. Massage helps increase blood flow in muscles and other tissues, and helps instill a sense of well-being in both patient and caregiver.

Light Massages

- Schedule light massages in the patient's daily routine.

- Schedule massages at convenient times during the day, such as when watching TV.

- Before getting out of bed in the morning and after an afternoon nap, give the patient a gentle warm-up stretch and massage.

- Massage hands and feet, neck and shoulders, upper and lower back, and arms and legs.

- Use the patient's favorite lotion to massage their hands.

- Massage the patient's feet in warm water. Then dry them and put on their socks.

Full-Body Massages

- Schedule a more thorough massage once or twice per week.
- Schedule full-body massages just before bathing times.
- Do the massage in bed or in a safe chair in the bath area.
- Use sesame or olive oil for deep massages.

Pets and Stuffed Animals

The patient may like to hold a stuffed animal or a plush toy. In case of anxiety, cuddling a stuffed animal can be soothing and may help the patient relax. Also, sitting next to pets such as dogs and cats or watching fish swim about inside a fish tank may reduce anxiety and help the patient focus on something new.

11 | GETTING TO COOPERATION

etting the patient to cooperate can be a challenge. In the early stage of dementia progression, the patient will likely resist giving up control and insists on managing their affairs on their own. In the middle stage, the patient may no longer understand what you want them to do. In the late stage, the patient may be unable to comply with your requests altogether.

- Over time, the patient will be less and less able to understand your words and ideas or how they relate to the issue at hand.

- Impaired impulse control means the patient will have difficulty negotiating the urge to do, or not do, something.

You usually can't reason with the patient because of impaired cognition and impulse control. However, with a little planning and creativity, you can often find ways to get their cooperation naturally and without the need for logic and explanation.

GETTING THE PATIENT TO GIVE UP CONTROL

It's walking a tightrope. If we intervene too early, we take away their self-confidence. And if we intervene too late, we risk accidents from which we may not be able to recover.

Whether the patient should continue to drive, manage their finances, or handle their medication on their own are common areas of contention during the early stage of dementia progression. Patients usually resist giving up control. They often insist that they are fully capable of managing their own affairs, well past the time when it is safe for them to do so.

To ensure that the patient's critical affairs are conducted safely, you'll have to find a way to take over managing them. You'll have to get the patient to let you take over, and to cooperate when you do. This requires skill and patience on your part so ensuring safety does not devolve into acrimony and conflict.

Why Patients Resist

Long before a diagnosis of dementia, patients may rely on notes and reminders to compensate for a failing memory. Notes and reminders become anchors to life and a way to hold on to events as they march on. Similarly, driving, cooking, work, and finances are anchors to a life that is familiar. Without anchors mooring one to firm ground, one is left twisting in the wind.

To give up control means to surrender. It means to give up autonomy, to be vulnerable to the unknown that is closing in on all sides, and to trust that someone will be there to anticipate and tend to your needs. It's a tall order because one who is falling tends instinctively to reach out, grasping, to keep from falling. To help someone give up control, you have to instill a sense of security and trust strong enough to overcome the instinct to hold on.

- Address the patient's anxiety. Assure them that you will be there for them and will take care of them. Ease their anxiety overall, rather than focusing on what you want them to give up.

- Ease the patient into giving up control. Initially, it may be enough just to keep an eye out for safety when they cook, drive, or handle finances.

- Add safeguards over time, as the need arises. Reduce their credit card spending limit, let them manage less critical medications such as vitamin or other supplements, and help them with the more difficult cooking tasks.

- Make it easy for the patient to give up control by doing it incrementally. It's a lot easier for someone to give up an inch today and another inch tomorrow, than it is to give it all up in one go.

Balancing Safety and Independence

Help maintain patient independence and self-esteem by letting them manage their own affairs for as long as they can. To keep them safe, keep a watchful eye and intervene when they can no longer perform tasks safely.

- Monitor the patient's performance over time. Since dementia is a degenerative condition, a patient who is able to drive, cook, or manage their finances today will likely not remain so for long.

- Patients' cognition fluctuates during the course of a day. The patient may be relatively safe and capable during the morning hours when they are well rested and relaxed. They may be less so in the afternoon, when they are tired or hungry.

How to Ask a Loved One to Give Up Control

Ideally, you'd want to get the patient to agree to let you take over a task for them. You can usually reason with a patient in the early stages of Alzheimer's disease and convince them that it is unsafe for them to drive, cook, or manage their finances. But, because they easily forget, you'll need to have this conversation with them again and again. With a patient suffering from frontotemporal dementia, reasoning is futile. Because of impaired reasoning, you cannot convince them of anything.

- Talk to the patient about the reasons why they should stop driving, managing their meds, or whatever. Describe your concerns regarding the physical and financial burdens that a mistake may inflict on the family.

- Suggest alternatives. Offer to help them cook, drive them wherever they need to go, or give them cash whenever they need it.

- Draw on authority figures, such as their doctor, the department of motor vehicles, and elders or family members that the patient respects. Get help from grandchildren or others for whom the patient has a soft spot and is more likely to agree to make a sacrifice.

- Do not expect the patient to yield with a single conversation. They may agree to give up one thing easily, while resisting to give up something else. Letting someone else manage their medication may be liberating, while not being able to drive may mean giving up their independence.

- If the patient reacts in an angry or aggressive way, postpone the discussion for another time, when they are calm and well rested. Anxiety and aggression can be made worse by the looming loss of independence.

- Face this problem with love and understanding. Express yourself with kindness and reassure the patient of your unconditional love and support. But insist that they let you take over critical tasks.

If All Else Fails

If you cannot get the patient to agree to let you take over a critical task, you'll have to take more drastic measures. Even if they do agree to relinquish control, additional measures can help reduce repeated arguments in the future.

- Hide car keys, tools, kitchen appliances, credit cards, medication, and so on.

- Disable the car, stove, appliances, and power tools.

- Distract the patient and redirect their attention with all the cleverness and trickery that you can muster.

Getting Past "No"

I wish I was the same person my wife married years ago, but I'm not. I wish I could travel, socialize with friends, or play with my grandchildren, but I can't. Holding myself together takes a lot of energy, more than I can muster. I'm exhausted. I cannot make simple decisions or hold a conversation with anyone. I feel the world drifting away, and feel helpless to stop it. I'm tired and lonely.

Over time, the patient will show less and less interest in engaging with life and those around them. This may be due to the fact that communication and social interaction are cognitively demanding exercises, which the patient may find utterly draining. Or, they may simply be lost as to what to say or do next, causing them to disengage. However, it is still important to try to engage with the patient and encourage them to interact with you.

- Try to communicate without exhausting the patient. Use short, simple sentences, and do not ask too many questions.

- Your interactions must be genuine, attentive, and generous. Don't expect the patient to communicate if you are busy with your cell phone or tablet, or are busy watching TV.

- Try different techniques to engage the patient. Do not be discouraged if an approach that worked yesterday does not work today. Be flexible and find new ways to connect.

Decoding "No"

People with dementia tend to answer questions with "no." Are you thirsty? No. Do you want some fruit? No. Do you need to go to the bathroom? No.

No is the default answer, one that requires the least amount of mental effort or consideration. To answer otherwise would require thinking about the question, evaluating its consequences, imagining what the world would be like as a result, and deciding whether it is something they would like to happen. It's an exhausting amount of mental processing, especially if the questions keep coming.

- Do not ask too many questions. Remember that the cognitive effort involved in processing and answering a question can be exhausting. Keep questions for when you really need an answer.

- Communicate by means that don't demand so much cognitive effort. Use touch, caress, simple sentences, and sweet words of comfort and love to connect with the patient.

- To ask a question or otherwise communicate with the patient, gently draw them out of their mental cocoon. Imagine you're trying to wake them up. Use a little touch and gentle caressing of the hands. Give their mind a bit of stimulation and a bit of time to warm up.

Getting Through With Finesse

My mom sleeps all the time. She stays up just long enough to eat her breakfast and an early lunch and then goes back to bed. We've tried delaying her lunch just to keep her up for an hour longer. But, she'd rather go to bed hungry than wait for her meal.

Boredom, apathy, and depression are common in dementia. The patient may seem like they're putting up walls, but they are not. Inactivity and lack of involvement in meaningful tasks can sap one's energy and motivation. When cognitive impairment is added to the mix, the smallest task can feel like an insurmountable barrier.

- Recognize the immense effort it takes for the patient to engage with anything. Do not give up trying to find ways to draw them out, but do so in thoughtful ways, matching your approach to their ability and energy levels.

- When the patient does not have the energy to engage with tasks, sometimes a hug or simple togetherness are the most effective ways to engage.

- Remember that engagement is not just about doing things. It's about being a part of something. Holding the patient's hands and caressing them, saying kind words, or just being together can help the patient be part of the life that is going on around them.

SEE ACTIONS THROUGH PATIENT'S EYES

We bought Mom a gold bracelet for her birthday. We got one with a latch that couldn't be easily opened so she wouldn't lose it. The next day, Mom wasn't wearing it. I asked her where her bracelet was. She didn't answer. "Where is your bracelet, Mom?" I asked again, and she pointed to the garbage bin. Inside the bin atop the pile of trash, I found the bracelet, in pieces.

To understand an action, consider the problem it's trying to solve and the mental processes behind the problem-solving effort. Cognitive impairment means that the patient often cannot find solutions that would be obvious to a healthy individual.

When cognitive processing is impaired, alternatives are not discovered, and consequences are not evaluated. The first thing that comes to mind is the only solution that is available, and the only course of action that is pursued. Any attempt to reason with the patient, or suggest alternatives, is in vain because they cannot keep track of what they're doing and carry a conversation with you at the same time.

- Do not take the action personally. It is simply the one solution that the patient has discovered to address a particular problem.

- Do not try to reason with the patient. If possible, go with the flow and fix later. If the patient wants to move a chair, help them move it, and later on return the chair to its proper place.

- Distract the patient by planting a different idea in their mind. Point to something nearby and ask them a question about it. Then dovetail with other questions that progressively lead the patient away from the original action.

Do Not Block or Respond With a "No"

Sooner or later, dementia begins to impair impulse control. The patient loses the ability to keep impulses in check, or to otherwise redirect and refocus their attention to something else. Eventually, there are no more requests, only demands, and whatever the patient wants, they want it right away.

- Impaired impulse control means that the patient cannot just stop wanting to do something. You'll have to find a way to redirect their attention instead.

- Impaired impulse control also makes it impossible for the patient to accept a "no", or respect that you cannot comply with their wishes.

- Do not start with a no, for example, "No, we don't have any ice cream," or "No ice cream before lunch." A response that starts with no is almost guaranteed to trigger an aggressive reaction.

- Instead, go with the flow and redirect. Start with a yes or okay followed by a redirect: "Yes, after we have lunch we'll go to your sister's," or "Okay, after our walk in the park we'll stop for ice cream."

BYPASSING FORCE WITH FLOW

We were late for our doctor's visit, and Mom was not cooperating. We finally had to forcibly get her dressed, then pick her up and carry her to the car.

There may be times when you'll have to physically force or restrain the patient to keep them from doing something dangerous or causing harm to themselves or others. With proper planning, however, such episodes should be rare to nonexistent. Given the patient's declining cognitive capacity, it is usually possible to find creative ways to distract and redirect the patient without having to resort to force.

Resorting to force is deeply destructive. Its physiological and psychological effects linger long afterwards, setting up the patient and caregiver for more conflict down the road. This is a vicious cycle, with each episode compounding the effects of the previous ones. Avoid it if at all possible because once it gets started, it's very hard to reset everyone's physiology back to baseline.

Plan Ahead

To do anything that involves the patient, you'll have to set the stage so they go along with the plan. Since you can't rely on words to make the patient see what you want to do and why, you'll have to rely on more subtle means to get their cooperation.

Remember that the patient faces a world of unknowns at every turn. They need to know why you want them to do something, yet they cannot understand your explanations. Since you can't explain what lies around the corner, you have to focus their attention on the next immediate step or distract them altogether.

- Start getting ready early. Give yourself plenty of time to work around obstacles that will invariably arise as you try to get the patient dressed and ready for the task.

- If the patient resists the next step, stop and try again, perhaps in another way. Forcing the patient over the next step will just set them up for greater resistance over the following step.

- Mind your own emotional state. If you are anxious about the traffic and arriving on time for an appointment, your anxiety will affect the patient, no matter how hard you try to hide it.

Use the Right Cues

If you try to force the patient, you'll trigger an automatic fight or flight response. If you overwhelm the patient with instructions, you'll trigger an aggressive response. Before you engage with the patient, think through the kind of response you'd like to bring about, then create a situation that naturally leads to the desired behavior. Lay out cues like breadcrumbs in front of the patient, in a way that invites them to follow the desired course of action. Take care to avoid situations that cue the patient otherwise.

I had to move the car out of the garage before Mom could get in on the passenger side. But, she stood too close to the car, making it impossible to safely move it. So I had her hold on to the handle of the door opening into the house. I moved the car and looked over, and she had disappeared. Inside the house, I found her all the way at the far end, rummaging through the bedroom closet.

It took me a while to figure out what had happened: the weight of her arm had turned the door handle, causing the door to open into the house, and cueing her to walk through. The empty living room had led her to the hallway, then to the stairs, the bedroom upstairs, and finally to the closet at the back of the bedroom. The closet was a dead-end, cueing her to the shelves, drawers, and boxes.

Now, I lock the door before having her hold on to the handle. When I come to fetch her a few second later, the door handle has fully turned under the weight of her arm, but she's still there holding on to it.

Use Distraction to Advantage

When the patient cannot follow your reasoning, they cannot cooperate with you. Even if they still understand words, they may have difficulty in staying with you long enough to get the gist of your meaning. So, instead of trying to keep them focused, use their distractibility to your advantage.

When we got home, Mom didn't want to remove her long winter coat. "Mom, come here, I want to show you something," I said, taking her hand and leading her to the living room. There, I pointed to the photos on the wall and, while she was waiting to see what I wanted to show her, I started to unbutton her coat from the top. It took a moment before she noticed that her top buttons were undone and started to button them up again. I continued to make my way down her coat until I reached the last button, then circled back to the top and quickly caught up to her, still working on the third or fourth button.

At this point I needed another distraction. "Hold this for me, Mom," I said, handing her a bulky remote control from the coffee table next to us. Then I handed her a second, and then a third remote. With her attention now consumed by the impossible task of managing three remotes with two hands, I finished unbuttoning her coat and began removing it. "Wait, wait..." she kept saying, bewildered as I slid her hands through the sleeves, taking care that she not let go of the remotes in the process. When I was done, I let her go, and she promptly disappeared into an adjoining room, still fumbling with the remotes. A moment later, she reemerged, empty handed, all eager and helpful. "Okay, tell me what you want to do," she said. I said something like, "I want you to kiss me on the cheek," and presented my cheek. Looking over her shoulder, I could see the three remotes on the edge of the bed in the other room. The coffee table had been right next to her, and still, she had gone all the way to the other room to unload the remotes.

Assess Risks Beforehand

The key to preventing conflict is looking ahead. It is much easier to bypass a potential problem, than rely on ingenuity to solve it. An ounce of prevention really is better than a pound of cure. And sometimes, prevention means forgoing the activity altogether.

Whenever you want to do something, such as go to the park, think through possible consequences. Can you handle the patient alone? Can the patient handle the stress, or will they respond with agitation or aggression?

- What if the patient needs to go to the bathroom?
- What if they wet or soil their pants?
- What if they refuse to leave the park to go home?
- What if they get agitated by the noise and the crowd?
- What if you get into a fender bender along the way?

Before setting off on an activity, think about why you are doing it. Is it for you or for the patient? If they become agitated or anxious, is it due to something within your control that you can fix, or is it because they really don't feel safe or comfortable?

PICK YOUR BATTLES

She had become outgoing and talkative. She berated relatives for all the slights and annoyances of the past. In family gatherings, she'd sing and dance. One time, I noticed she was wearing mismatched socks, but she didn't care.

There will be many times when the patient wants to do something that, for one reason or another, you find objectionable. If you try to intervene each and every time, you'll create a life that is full of argument, agitation, and calamity for both you and the patient. Instead, gauge the situation and intervene only if the patient is about to do something that is unsafe or dangerous. So, if the patient wants to eat with their hands, let them be; if they want to get something off their chest, let them do it; but if they want to leave home in the middle of the night, find ways to distract them.

12 | Nutrition and Hydration

Over the course of dementia, it becomes increasingly difficult to ensure that the patient is receiving adequate nutrition. In the early stages, indulgence, inactivity, and unhealthy food choices may lead to excessive weight gain and obesity, while in the later stages, weight loss, malnutrition, and dehydration become more dominant health risks. Reduced appetite, forgetfulness, restlessness, and anxiety create barriers to getting enough food. Eventually swallowing problems, decreased mobility, and becoming bedridden make adequate nutrition even more difficult. Some 30 to 40 percent of patients with dementia may experience clinically significant weight loss during the course of their illness.

Plan a Healthy Diet

He constantly complained of hunger, and minutes after eating, wanted something to eat again. She wouldn't eat, and would say she had already eaten.

The amount of food and fluids that an individual needs varies according to the season, and their daily activity, weight, and metabolism. A simple formula, such as 2000 calories per day, is not suitable for everyone. Also, conditions such as high blood pressure or diabetes may require special dietary considerations. If necessary, consult a nutritionist.

- Plan a balanced diet based on the patient's needs and the kinds of food they like.

- Incorporate elements of the Mediterranean diet, with fruits, vegetables (generally steamed or boiled), oily fish, cereals, and legumes. The Mediterranean diet has been shown to enhance cognitive function.

- Adopt the nutritionally improved food guide pyramid, with emphasis on leafy greens, legumes, nuts and seeds, vegetables, fruits, oily fish, and eggs.

- Use ingredients such as carrots, cauliflowers, squash, tomatoes, chickpeas, beans, lentils, and fruits, as well as low-fat dairy and low-fat proteins like poultry and fish.

- Include nuts and seeds. Serve a handful of unsalted nuts as snack, or slice/grind them and add to other foods such as salad, yogurt, and smoothies.

- Keep consumption of saturated fats low. Reduce consumption of butter, margarine, high-fat dairy products, and fatty meats.

- Avoid sugar, soft drinks, and sweets, as much as possible.

- Reduce salt intake. Remove the saltshaker from the table so the patient does not use too much salt on their food.

- Ensure adequate hydration. Make sure the patient gets about six to eight glasses of fluids properly staggered throughout each day.

- Do not medicate the patient on your own, and do not put them on vitamin and other food supplements without consulting their doctor. The ingredients in these products may not be compatible with the patient's underlying health issues or their medications.

Reduce the Risk of Malnutrition

When dementia hit, my mom weighed 99 pounds. She has lost a lot of weight since then, although I don't know how much because there's no way to weigh her. She eats very little, and if we beg and cajole her to eat more, she invariably throws up afterwards. I worry that when swallowing problems start, her eating will get a lot worse.

Excessive weight loss and malnutrition are problems that many patients and caregivers will eventually face. These problems are gateways to further complications down the road and must be dealt with as soon as possible.

- Cook the patient's food well so the ingredients are not tough and do not require much chewing. Cut meat, poultry, and fish into small bite-sized pieces.

- Watch for swallowing problems. They will become more severe over time. At some point, you'll have to blend the patient's food for easier swallowing.

- Watch the patient's appetite closely to prevent unwanted weight loss. Encourage them to eat enough by preparing meals that they like.

- Increase the number of meals and snacks, and reduce the amount of each serving to keep the patient's weight balanced.

- Allow plenty of time for each meal or snack so the patient has adequate time to finish their food.

- Evaluate the reasons for any loss of appetite and try to fix them. Do the patient's dentures fit properly? Does the patient have tooth or gum infection? Is the patient constipated? Are they suffering from a urinary tract infection? Is the loss of appetite related to a change in medication?

- To increase appetite, try appetizing syrups. If the patient cannot eat enough to receive all the nutrients that they need, you may augment their diet with nutritional supplements or meal replacement products specifically designed for this purpose. Consult your doctor or pharmacist.

A Taste for Sweets

My father has developed a sweet tooth. He has an insatiable appetite for sugary sodas, candy, and ice cream. The other day he emptied an entire bowl of candy in a few minutes. He has gained weight and has lost mobility. I'm at a loss as to how to control his appetite for sweets.

In some types of dementia, such as frontotemporal dementia (FTD), the patient develops a sweet tooth. This is often the result of impaired impulse control, where the patient loses the ability to keep impulses in check or to redirect and refocus their attention to something else.

- Impaired impulse control means that the patient cannot just stop wanting some sweets. You'll have to find a way to redirect their attention instead.

- Do not argue. If the patient complains that they haven't had any ice cream, showing them empty wrappers won't help.

- Use activities to distract the patient and to buy time. Take the patient for a walk in the park, with the promise of ice cream when you get to your destination.

- Hide sugary foods and sweets, but don't deny the patient one of the few of life's remaining pleasures. Instead, stay alert to ensure that their consumption remains moderate.

- Make sweets a regular part of your daily routine. When serving sweets, bring a reasonable serving for each person present. Do not place a bowl full of sweets on the table for people to serve themselves.

- Instead of sweets, leave low-calorie snacks like butter-free popcorn, and vegetables like carrots, cauliflower, and broccoli on the table within easy reach. Use low-fat yogurt as a dip.

Rummaging through closets, Mom had discovered her stash of candy, had filled her pockets to the brim, and was already eating one. She looked so cute in her blue sweater vest, with both pockets and one cheek bulging with candy. I asked her what she was eating. She said, "Candy," and gave me one. I put the candy in my pocket, out of view, and said, "Give me one, too." She handed me another one. I hid the candy and asked again, and she gave me another and then another, until my pockets were full and hers were empty. It was heartbreaking how easy it was to trick her. I asked if she had any more in her pockets. She searched and pulled out one last piece. I said, "Give me that one, too." She said, "Then I won't have any left for myself." My heart ached as I asked again, gently as before, "Give me one, too, Mommy," and she gave me her last piece.

Staying Hydrated

When water loss through sweat, urine, and evaporation is not compensated through adequate water intake, dehydration begins to set in. Unlike malnutrition, which may take days and weeks to develop, dehydration can set in within hours. Dehydration is associated with reduced cognitive function, lower physical performance, and degraded immune function. Confusion, irritability, anxiety, fatigue, constipation, and an increased susceptibility to infections such as urinary tract infection, are possible complications. Severe dehydration can lead to kidney failure and cardiac arrest.

How Much Water Do We Need?

- An individual typically needs six to eight glasses of fluids a day. Excess weight, physical activity, and warm weather all increase the amount of fluids a person needs.

- Diuretics, anti-histamines, laxatives, and many other drugs increase the rate of water loss from the body, resulting in a higher risk of dehydration.

- Diarrhea, vomiting, and fever may cause significant water loss from the body, increasing the risks of severe dehydration. Severe dehydration is serious and requires immediate medical attention.

Symptoms of Dehydration

The best gauge of hydration status is the amount and color of urine. The urine of a well-hydrated person is mostly clear or light yellow in color, and odorless. With dehydration, urine volume is reduced and its color turns darker. Symptoms of dehydration include:

- Decreased urine volume

- Dark-yellow urine

- Headache

- Constipation

- Muscle cramps

- Dry mouth

- Drowsiness

- Fatigue.

Severe Dehydration

Severe dehydration is dangerous and can quickly escalate to a life-threatening condition. It is associated with low blood volume, inadequate electrolytes, and heart and kidney stress. If not treated promptly, it can lead to kidney failure, cardiac arrest, coma, or death.

Symptoms of severe dehydration include:

- Severe reduction in urine volume

- Dark-colored urine

- Dry skin – when you pinch the skin on the back of the hand lightly with two fingers, it takes longer than usual to return to its original appearance

- Clammy hands and feet

- Dizziness and confusion

- Low blood pressure

- Rapid breathing

- Rapid, weak pulse.

Preventing Dehydration

Dementia patients may not notice that they are thirsty, may forget to drink water, or may be unable to communicate that they need water. As swallowing problems and incontinence begin to appear on the scene, caregivers may unwittingly reduce the amount of fluids they serve to patients, and patients may hesitate, or refuse, to drink.

- Don't wait for the patient to ask for water. By the time they feel thirsty, dehydration has already set in.

- Schedule fluids at specific times in the patient's daily schedule. With a proper daily hydration schedule, you can ensure that the patient is receiving the amount of fluids that they need.

- Keep track of the patient's hydration status in the daily log. Include the number and timing of bathroom visits, the amount of urine output, and its color. Adjust their scheduled fluid intake based on these logs so the daily schedule reflects the amount of fluids that the patient really needs.

- Don't be alarmed if the patient's urine is darker immediately after waking up in the morning. That is normal because they haven't had anything to drink overnight. However, do serve fluids bright and early after waking up to make up for it.

- Take care to not unwittingly reduce the patient's fluid intake for fear of incontinence or swallowing problems. Rely on the daily schedule and the daily log to keep your memory of the fluids served firmly in contact with reality.

- Carefully monitor the patient's fluid intake in all seasons because dehydration can occur even in cold weather.

How to Increase Fluid Intake

It may be hard to entice the patient to drink enough water. Fortunately, hydration is not limited to the amount of water one drinks. Many foods, especially fruits and vegetables, contain plenty of water:

	Water (%)
Cucumber	96
Tomato	94
Watermelon	92
Grape	92
Mellon	90
Apple	84

How you serve foods and fluids influences the patient's fluid consumption. Think creatively and serve food and fluids in ways that entice the patient to consume it.

Tap Into Extra Sources of Water

- Add a few strawberries or other fruits to breakfast cereals.
- Add a few lettuce leaves and a slice of tomato to sandwiches.
- Serve soups that contain lots of water, such as chicken and vegetable soups.
- Serve frozen yogurt with a few strawberries and other fruits for added flavor.

Add Flavor to Water

- Flavor water with a few drops of rose water, peppermint extract, or lemon juice.
- Put a slice of lemon in a glass of water.
- Serve natural fruit juices.

- Limit the consumption of caffeine and sweetened beverages.

Serve Water in Interesting Ways

- Use colored glasses that are easier for the patient to see.

- Use beautiful glasses that are saved for special occasions. They can be interesting to the patient and may motivate them to drink the contents.

- Add a lemon wedge to the edge of the glass to increase its appeal.

13 | MEAL TIMES AND SWALLOWING PROBLEMS

A t the beginning stages of dementia, eating and drinking continue much as before. The patient recognizes when they are hungry or thirsty and knows where to obtain food or water. This period of relative independence does not last long. Soon, problems with memory, judgment, and decision-making begin to affect everything, from meal planning and preparation to remembering to eat, or even recognizing that they are hungry or thirsty.

Initially, the patient will need assistance with simple things, like preparing their meals, reminding them that it's time to eat, and encouraging them to finish their food. They may need more time to consume their meals, may need someone to cut their food, may prefer to eat by hand, and may spill their food. They may need their meals served in order, for example, salad first, then the main course, followed by dessert.

Over time, eating and drinking become more challenging. Eventually the patient will be unable to eat on their own and will depend on their caregiver for assistance with every bite.

MEAL TIMES

My wife's dementia came on early and progressed rapidly. She lost the ability to use a knife and fork a long time ago, and soon couldn't even eat with her hands. She loved pizza, and we'd go out together, and I'd feed her. In the beginning, people would nod approvingly at how well I cared for my wife. Over time, she deteriorated and lost a lot of weight. Now, people pat me on the back for taking such good care of my mother.

In the early stage of dementia, patients typically do not need a special diet and are able to have their meals together with the rest of the family. Over time, however, they gradually lose the ability to join the rest of the family at meal times and will need separate mealtime planning.

Meal times are cognitively challenging. The variety of foods within reach, the plates, cups, and utensils and the dilemma of how to use each, the number of people at the table and the various threads of conversation going on, all add up to a cognitive load that can be overwhelming for the patient. As a result, the patient may make more mistakes than usual, may spill their food, may become restless or agitated, or may stop eating altogether.

The handling of utensils, cutting one's food, and otherwise navigating one's dinner plate involve fine hand-eye and motor coordination, which requires considerable processing in the brain. With advancing dementia, what the patient intends to do may not translate to the right movements of their hands and fingers. As a result, the patient will progressively need more help at meal times.

Make Meal Times Easier

Sooner or later, the patient will need more help at meal times. They may fill their spoon with food but forget to put it in their mouth. They may forget how to use their utensils, and may be confused by the various condiments and spices on the table. They may have difficulty deciding which food to choose from among the variety available on the table.

- Set the table in the simplest possible way. Remove all sauces, spices, salt and pepper from the table.

- Eliminate distractions. Turn off the TV and avoid loud conversations. If necessary, serve the patient's meals in a quiet room, with only the caregiver present.

- Serve the patient's food in sequence, for example, first serve their salad or soup, and then bring the main dish to the table. To prevent overeating, serve their meals in a specific plate or bowl, and bring it to the table to prevent seconds.

- Serve the patient's meals in brightly colored plates and cups, using colorful utensils. Red plates usually work the best. In one study, patients eating from red plates consumed about 25 percent more food than those eating from white plates. Use plates that are a different color than the tablecloth or the food itself.

- Use deeper plates to serve the patient's meals. Deep plates make it easier to pick up pieces of food or fill a spoon with the help of the plate's edge.

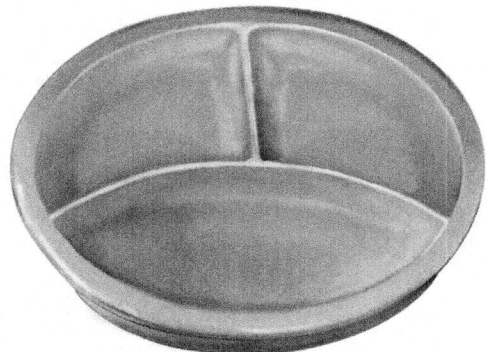

Figure 13.1 Deep plate with compartments.
The walls make it easier to pick up pieces of food.

- Alternatively, use fancy plates, cups, and silverware that the patient might have kept for special occasions. Serve liquids in interesting glasses to make it more likely that the patient will drink them.

- Place their plate on a tablemat to prevent it from sliding around and falling.

Prolong Patient Independence

Patients' independence impacts their self-confidence and their quality of life. Let the patient eat on their own and at their own pace, even if they happen to spill their food or eat by hand.

- Serve the patient's meals with food already cut into small, bite-sized pieces, or serve it as a sandwich for easier handling. If they prefer to eat their meal by hand, let them.

- Make sure the food being served is not so hot as to burn the patient. The patient is likely not able to remember to watch out for their plate or food being too hot.

- Be flexible. If the patient doesn't want to eat a specific food, don't force them. If they want to eat one or two types of food every day, that's okay, too. Just make sure that their meal is balanced and meets dietary recommendations.

- Allow plenty of time for each meal or snack so the patient does not feel rushed.

- If they spill their food a lot, use a long apron to keep their clothes clean. Fold the bottom of the apron and sew the edges to create a trough to collect food debris.

- Serve the patient's meals in a place where it is easy to wash and clean afterwards.

- Treat the patient with kindness and respect. Do not reprimand them and never talk down to them or treat them like a child.

SAFE FEEDING

My mother is still mobile and recognizes everyone. But, she eats too fast and does not swallow completely before taking the next bite. Soon enough, her mouth gets full, and the whole process grinds to a halt.

With progressing dementia, eating and drinking grow more challenging. The patient may take a bite and then forget to chew it, or may chew but then forget to swallow. Before swallowing the previous bite, they may take another bite, until their mouth is full and they're unable to swallow. This is called food pocketing, and when it happens, the only solution is to empty their mouth so the swallowing process can restart.

Food pocketing is dangerous. It interferes with the swallowing process and may lead to food aspiration, with food entering the windpipe and the lungs. This usually causes severe coughing, and can lead to lung infection, aspiration pneumonia, or even choking and suffocation.

General Procedure for Safe Feeding

- Food pocketing is more likely if the patient eats on their own. It is critical for the patient's safety that you stay present during meal times and monitor the process carefully.

- Serve meals in a quiet environment and allow plenty of time so the patient doesn't feel rushed. This is especially important during the late stage of dementia, when the patient has difficulty swallowing.

- Eliminate distractions so the patient can concentrate on eating or drinking. Turn off the TV, and ask others to be quiet and not walk around the area where the patient is being fed.

- Sit the patient perfectly upright and tilt their head slightly forward. This posture helps to keep the windpipe closed during swallowing.

- Make sure the patient has finished swallowing the previous bite before taking the next bite. If they get stuck with too much food in their mouth, you'll have to empty their mouth before the process can restart.

- In case of severe coughing, the patient may throw up. Stay calm, lean the patient forward, and let them vomit. Then wipe their mouth and tongue with a wet oral sponge swab. Before feeding them anything again, including any fluids, make sure their mouth is completely empty.

When the Patient Does Not Cooperate

My mom refuses to open her mouth to be fed. We've had to force her mouth open to feed her.

Never force the patient's mouth open. You may harm them physically and emotionally. Instead, try to find the root cause of the problem and address that. If the problem has developed recently, it's likely that some change in routine or in the patient's condition has triggered it. Look for changes in medication, room, residence, or caregiver. Also, consider the possibility of new or recurring conditions such as constipation, urinary tract infection, tooth or gum inflammation, or other illnesses such as cold or flu.

FORGETTING TO SWALLOW

At some point, the patient may chew their food but forget to swallow it. Usually, it's not too difficult to cue the process to resume.

- Calmly remind the patient to swallow. Gently touch their lips, chin, and cheeks to help activate the swallowing reflex.

- Bring an empty spoon to their lips as if feeding them the next morsel of food. If they open their mouth, put the empty spoon in their mouth. This may help restart the process and get them to swallow the food already in their mouth.

- Give them a small amount of a different kind of food that is incongruous to what they were eating. A bit of ice cream, jam, or yogurt may help trigger the swallowing reflex.

- Do not use a spoon or fork as a lever to force the patient's mouth open. Such tactics are stressful and dangerous, and may injure their teeth and gums. It also increases the chances of food or liquids entering their windpipe.

Using a Suction Device

If you are unable to restart the swallowing process, the next option is to empty the patient's mouth. You can use a suction device to remove any pocketed food or liquid from their mouth.

- A suction device is a portable unit similar to the device dentists use to clear saliva from a patient's mouth. You can purchase a portable suction device from medical supply stores.

- Choose a model that works with electricity from a wall outlet as well as rechargeable batteries. Follow the manufacturer's recommendation to keep the batteries fully charged and ready to go at all times. When you go out with the patient, take the suction device with you.

- When you are unable to cue the swallowing process to resume using the above techniques, use the suction device to empty the patient's mouth completely before continuing with the feeding.

- Patients will usually start to eat and swallow normally again after their mouth has been cleared.

WHEN SWALLOWING IS COMPROMISED

Swallowing involves complex neuromuscular coordination among a number of organs to allow food and fluids to pass from the mouth into the esophagus, safely bypassing the windpipe. A slight impairment anywhere in the process may result in food or fluids going the wrong way and into the windpipe, causing severe coughing.

- Watch for signs of swallowing issues early in the course of dementia progression. If necessary, consult a speech therapist sooner, rather than later, to evaluate any swallowing issues.

- Prepare yourself for a choking emergency by learning the Heimlich maneuver. Check for classes at your local hospital or community center.

The Danger of Food Aspiration

Swallowing problems tend to develop in the late stage of dementia progression, and sometimes as early as the middle stage. As the patient loses the ability to chew their food completely or swallow it safely, the possibility of food or fluids entering their windpipe grows more likely.

The entry of food and fluids into the windpipe is usually accompanied by severe coughing. Even if the patient is able to cough strongly enough to expel the errant food from their windpipe, some of the food may still end up in their lungs (food aspiration), which may result in lung infection (aspiration pneumonia).

Managing swallowing problems is a primary concern for caregivers because severe coughing is highly stressful, to the point that the patient may refuse to eat and drink altogether.

Puree Meals

Eventually, the patient will be unable to chew and swallow regular foods. At that point, there will be no choice but to puree their meals.

- Thoroughly cook beans, peas, and other solids to make chewing and swallowing easy and to postpone having to switch completely to pureed meals.

- Use a home blender or food processor to puree food to a consistency similar to yogurt. Pureed food does not require any chewing, is easier to swallow, and is less likely to end up in the patient's windpipe or lungs.

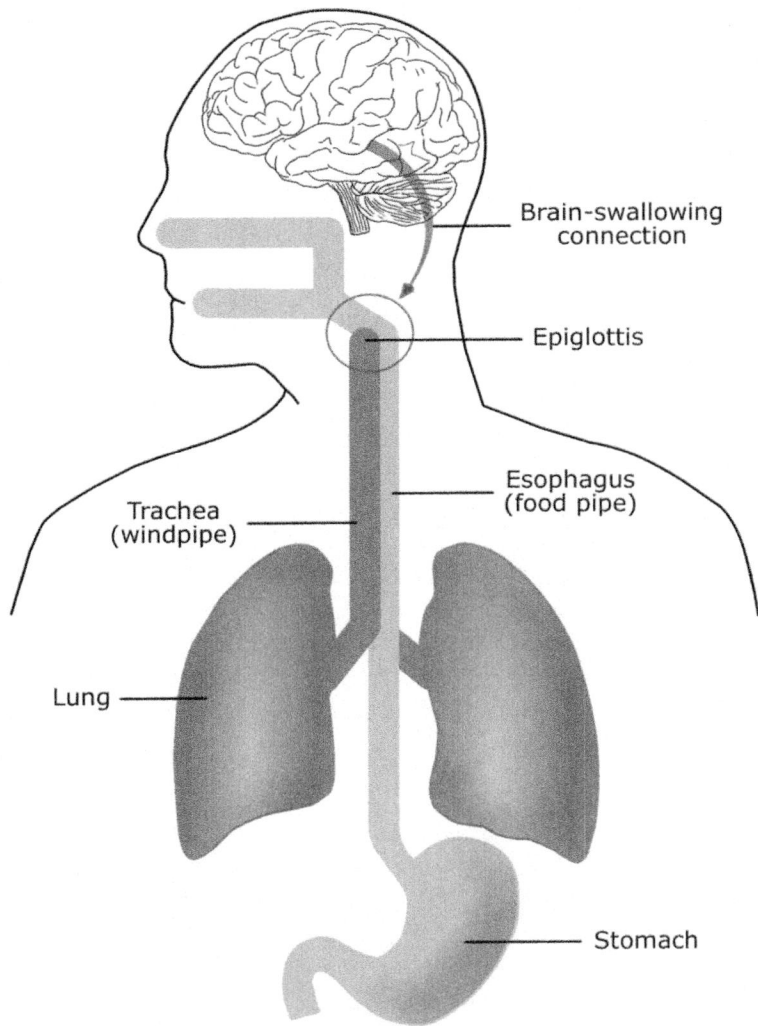

Figure 13.2 The swallowing mechanism.
The epiglottis directs traffic to the stomach or the lungs.

Thicken Liquids

Swallowing problems impair the patient's ability to drink fluids also. This time, the difficulty is due to the liquids being too thin, which makes it easy for the liquid to find its way into the patient's windpipe and lungs.

- Use food and beverage thickeners to thicken fluids, including drinking water. You can use commercial thickeners, or make your own using cornstarch.

- When preparing liquids, add just enough thickener to get the liquid to the needed consistency (see below). Add a little mint or sugar to make it more palatable and reduce the taste of starch.

- Initially, liquids need to be thickened just a little, similar to the consistency of syrup in canned fruits. But, over time, more thickening will become necessary. Eventually, the patient may need liquids at a consistency similar to that of honey or yogurt to be able to swallow safely.

When the Patient Cannot Drink From a Cup

At some point, drinking from a cup may become impractical, as the patient will have difficulty controlling the amount of liquid they take in with each sip. To prevent aspiration, you may use a syringe to serve liquids to the patient one sip at a time, typically 5CCs per sip. Alternatively, you may spoon-feed liquids to the patient.

What to Do About Phlegm

> *My wife coughs when she eats or drinks, sometimes very hard. I puree her food and I do not add any seasoning. She has a lot of phlegm accumulating in her throat, to the point that she cannot breathe comfortably.*

Swallowing problems are often accompanied by excess saliva, mucus, or phlegm building up in the mouth or throat. To reduce chest congestion, ask your doctor to prescribe a mucolytic syrup.

A useful procedure to dislodge phlegm from lungs and air canal is lung physiotherapy. Follow the procedure below several times a day:

- While the patient is sitting in a chair or on the toilet, lean them forward and, with your hand cupped, strike the patient's upper back several times, not too hard, and not too soft.

- Start easy at the beginning until you find the right level of force. Take care to not strike so hard as to cause discomfort in the patient. When done right, the patient seems quite at ease, with no sign of discomfort from the procedure.

- Practice on a healthy individual to find the right balance between hard and soft, and fine tune the shape of your cupped hand and the tension in your arm and shoulder. Make sure that you do not inflict pain on a helpless patient who is unable to communicate their discomfort to you.

WHEN THE PATIENT REFUSES TO EAT

My husband can no longer swallow his food and meds and chokes all the time. His doctor recommended that we surgically install a subcutaneous feeding tube in his stomach and feed him through that. But my son disagrees. I don't know what to do.

In the late stage of dementia, even a small amount of food or liquid may lead to severe coughing or suffocation. Eventually, the patient may become unable to swallow any food or liquids, and may refuse to eat or drink altogether.

At this stage, tube feeding through the nose or through a subcutaneous tube directly into the stomach may be the only remaining options. Whether to prolong the patient's life with such methods is one of the most difficult decisions confronting the family in the late stage. The one overriding factor should remain, as always, the best interests of the patient.

If the patient's wishes are known, these decisions will be a lot easier and less contentious. It is best to discuss end-of-life options early on, when the patient is still able to consider their options and articulate their wishes. They may request that all means be used to keep them alive, or may decide that they do not wish their life prolonged through such methods, or when no quality of life remains.

Eventually, there will come a time when the patient's organs begin to shut down as end-of-life draws near. This process may take days or weeks, during which the patient's food and fluid intake tapers off. Although it may be tempting to try to delay the inevitable by resorting to intravenous means to deliver nutrients to the patient's body, one should not lose sight of the fact that such interventions at this stage are quite stressful to the body as it undergoes its natural process of shutdown at the end of life.

14 | DRUG SAFETY

Oone of the early challenges after a diagnosis of dementia is to get the patient to hand over the task of managing their medications. Once they do, however, the work is just beginning. For most patients, the variety of their meds, along with their dosage and timing, makes it hard to keep track of them all and administer them at the right times and in the right amounts. On top of that, you'll have the added challenge of caring for a loved one who is growing increasingly vulnerable to mistakes, and progressively less able to cooperate with you.

GETTING THE PATIENT TO TAKE THEIR MEDS

She wouldn't take her meds. We'd hand her the pills, and she'd throw them. We'd ask, beg, and cajole her to let us put the pills in her mouth. She'd keep the pills under her tongue and then spit them out.

If the patient resists or otherwise acts stubbornly during medication times, remember that they're not doing so to create trouble. They may have difficulty swallowing their medication, may not like its taste, may not understand what you're asking of them, or may find the whole process anxiety provoking. Often, with a little creativity, you can redirect their behavior and get them to cooperate.

- Do not insist that the patient take their meds right then and there. If they refuse to take their meds, just leave it for a few moments and then try again.

- Change the atmosphere by recounting a happy anecdote. Use simple questions to help the patient engage with the story. Remain calm and cheerful to change their mood.

- Ask grandchildren or others dear to the patient for help in administering medications.

- Think of something that the patient enjoys, like going to the park or having a favorite sweet, and promise it to them if they take their medication.

Helping the Patient Understand

The patient will gradually lose the ability to understand conversations, and will need more time to process and respond to what is being asked of them. When administering medications, use simple words and short sentences. Pause after each sentence to give the patient time to comprehend what you are saying and to comply with your request.

1. Show the patient the pill and say: "This is your blood pressure medication." Then pause for a moment. Repeat the sentence, if necessary.

2. Bring the pill closer and say: "Put it in your mouth." Pause for a moment again. Repeat the sentence, if necessary.

3. If the patient does not take the pill, stand silent for a few moments. Use facial gestures that convey the plea: "Would you do it for me, please?" They will likely comply.

4. Once the pill is in the patient's mouth, hand them a glass of water. Pause for a moment and then say: "Drink water to swallow the pill."

SWALLOWING DIFFICULTIES

Over time, swallowing difficulties and the risk of food or medicine going the wrong way make the process of feeding or administering medication a difficult and hazardous exercise.

- Eliminate all distractions. Turn off the TV and the radio. Advise others not to come and go where the patient is being given their medication.

- Rely less on talk and more on gestures to convey your requests to the patient.

- To make swallowing easier, try administering meds with pureed food, thick yogurt, or ice cream instead of water.

- To help with swallowing, tilt the patient's head slightly forward. This helps close their windpipe and guide food and medication in the right path.

Helping the Patient to Swallow

In later stages of dementia progression, administering food and medication must proceed with simple verbal cues, and via triggering reflexes and other automatic behaviors.

1. Approach the patient with a bowl of yogurt and their medication. Let the patient see you approaching and process what is happening.

2. Fill the spoon with yogurt and put the pill over it. Bring the spoon to the patient's mouth. Hold the spoon near the patient's mouth until they open their mouth.

3. If the patient does not open their mouth, touch their lips gently with the spoon. You can open your own mouth to mimic the action so the patient reacts by opening theirs.

4. Sometimes the patient opens their mouth to receive the food and medication but then forgets to swallow. You may be able

to trigger the swallowing reflex by gently touching their chin, throat, and cheeks.

5.   If the patient still does not swallow, feed them a small spoon of ice cream or other food with a completely different taste and texture than what they have in their mouth.

6.   Never use a spoon or other utensils as a lever to force open the patient's mouth. This will cause pain and stress, and may injure the patient's lips, teeth, and gums.

7.   Throughout the process, inform the patient about what you are doing at each step using simple, short sentences. Do so even if they are not able to respond to you verbally.

If the Patient Vomits

Some medications, if not swallowed quickly, will dissolve in the mouth and leave behind a bad taste or texture, and may cause nausea and vomiting.

- If the patient throws up, do not panic. Keep them upright and lean them forward. Let them vomit. Then, make sure their mouth is completely empty.

- If you are sure that the medication has been completely thrown up, repeat that dose. Otherwise, do not give the patient another dose of the same medication at this time.

Crushing Meds Into a Powder

In the late stage of dementia progression, it may become impossible for the patient to swallow any pills or capsules. You'll have very limited options in dealing with this situation.

- One alternative is to use the liquid form of the medication, if one is available. Ask your doctor to prescribe the medication in liquid form.

- Another alternative is to crush the meds into a powder and mix it with food. But before doing so, be sure to consult with your doctor or pharmacist. Some meds require a specific mode of delivery, such as extended release capsules. Powdering such medications will interfere with their intended dosage, and may lead to drug interactions or other unexpected results.

REDUCING MEDICATION RISKS

Dementia presents its own set of risks and challenges when it comes to medication safety. The variety of meds one has to take makes mistakes more likely, and the type of meds involved makes forgetting to take a dose or taking it twice more dangerous.

- Psychotropic drugs affect brain chemistry and function. Taking less or more than the prescribed dose may have adverse effects, such as a loss in cognitive capacity, hallucination, or psychosis.

- Patients often take additional medications to control conditions such as hypertension and diabetes, and face a correspondingly higher risk of drug interactions and side effects.

- Dementia patients tend to be older and therefore more vulnerable to drug side effects. They may experience side effects more often and more severely.

- Most patients with dementia end up having swallowing difficulties. Simple approaches, such as crushing meds and mixing them with food, may prove harmful or even dangerous, as some drugs are not meant to be crushed.

Practice Drug Safety

- Do not medicate the patient on your own, and do not stop or start medications without prior consultation with their doctor. Many medications, prescription and over-the-counter, work by altering brain chemistry, including suppressing certain types of neurotransmitters. This may make them unsuitable for dementia patients.

- Do not crush any medication without consulting with your doctor or pharmacist. Crushing may interfere with the medication or its dosage, or may make it more susceptible to interaction with other drugs.

- Keep all medications in a safe and locked place to prevent misuse. Keep medications out of reach of the patient. Discard medications that are no longer needed or have expired.

- Keep alcohol, tobacco products, and other drugs out of view and out of reach. In case of substance dependency, give the patient a set amount at specific times, based on your doctor's instructions.

Starting the Patient On a New Drug

My mom has insomnia. Her doctor prescribed medication to help her sleep, but the drugs have caused problems in her behavior. She is confused, wants to sleep, but she cannot.

If your doctor prescribes medication to control a behavioral issue, follow the doctor's instructions carefully and be on the lookout for unwanted side effects. A typical procedure for starting the patient on a new prescription is as follows:

- Start the patient on one new medication at a time. In case of a change in dosage, change the dosage for one drug at a time. This way, in case of a bad side effect, you'll know which drug or dosage change is the likely culprit.

- Discuss any side effects with the doctor who prescribed the medication. Many of these complications may last only for a short while, while others may necessitate a change in medication or dosage.

- Psychotropic drugs may take up to two weeks to show their full effect. If you do not see any benefit after about two weeks, your doctor may change the medication or its dosage.

- Often, finding the appropriate drug to control a challenging behavioral problem may involve some trial and error.

Weaning the Patient Off of Unnecessary Drugs

Some medications, such as antibiotics, are prescribed for a specific period of time, while others, such as blood pressure medications and certain dementia drugs, are prescribed for use indefinitely. In practice, however, even long-term meds often run their course and should be discontinued eventually.

- When your doctor prescribes a new drug, make sure you understand how long the new meds are to be administered.

- Each time you visit your doctor, ask them if you should continue with the previous meds. If a drug is no longer necessary or effective, your doctor may reduce its dosage or stop it altogether.

- Do not stop a medication on your own, and do not change its dosage without prior consultation with your doctor.

- If your doctor decides to discontinue a drug or change its dosage, follow the doctor's instructions carefully. Many medications require their dosage to be reduced gradually over a period of time before they can be stopped safely.

Getting the patient to take their meds is often stressful for both the patient and their caregiver. Reducing the number of meds, or otherwise simplifying the patient's medication regimen, can help reduce acrimony and conflict, and improve quality of life for all involved.

MEDICATION SCHEDULE

The best way to stay on top of the patient's medication is to keep an up-to-date medication schedule, similar to the sample schedule of Figure 14.1. Include all of their prescribed medications and over-the-counter dietary supplements, as well as any pertinent information regarding each. Keep the schedule up to date, complete and accurate, and update it with any and all changes immediately.

- Write the exact name of the medication in the first column. Identify medications by name and not by appearance or color, since different medications may have similar shapes and colors.

- Next to the name of the medication, record the name of the prescribing doctor. In case of any side effects or issues, you'll know right away which doctor to contact.

- Record the date when the patient started taking the medication.

- Record the dosage and timing of the meds in the next two columns. Make sure to administer the medication exactly as ordered by the doctor.

- In the remaining columns, record any changes to the prescription, date of the change, and the name of the prescribing doctor, respectively. This information can help you monitor the impact of recent changes in medications.

Some caregivers prefer to update their medication list in pencil so they can make changes by erasing old entries and writing new changes in their place. But, doing so erases information that may come in handy in the future. A better approach would be to maintain the medication schedule in ink so you keep a history of changes. The historical information may prove helpful in deciphering unwanted changes in the patient's behavior and condition in the future.

You may prefer to keep the medication schedule on your computer or smartphone so you can update it easily and make backups to preserve a complete history.

Drug Name	Doctor	Date Started	Dose	Admin Time	Changes	Change Date	Doctor

Figure 14.1 Medication schedule

When Going to the Doctor

Make sure that each doctor treating the patient is aware of all the prescription and over-the-counter drugs the patient is currently taking.

- Whenever you visit a doctor, bring along the up-to-date medication schedule for them to review. The medication schedule helps the doctor make a more informed decision about any necessary changes to the patient's drug regimen.

- Inform your doctor about any allergies and side effects that the patient has experienced as a result of past medications.

- Inform your doctor of any alcohol, tobacco, or other substance dependency, so your doctor can adjust the patient's medication or its timing to reduce the risks of drug interactions.

- If your doctor prescribes new medication, make sure you understand how long the new meds are to be administered, their potential side effects, and possible interactions with any medication currently being taken by the patient.

- Ask your doctor if any of the patient's current medications can be reduced or eliminated. If so, make sure you understand the new dosage and timing for weaning the patient off of a drug.

- If the patient has difficulty swallowing, ask the doctor if the medication being prescribed is available in liquid form. If not, is it okay to crush the medication and mix it with food?

KEEPING MEDS ORGANIZED

The patient's medication regimen can be complex, making it difficult to keep track of and administer medication safely. To make it easier, separate the process of organizing and preparing meds from the hustle and bustle of daily caregiving.

Medication boxes make the process of administering meds easier and less error-prone by separating the preparation of the medication from their daily administration to the patient.

Medication Box

The best way to organize the patient's medications is to use medication boxes with seven compartments, one compartment for each day of the week. You'll need a separate box for each serving time, for example, one box for morning meds, one for noon, and a separate box for evening. Be sure to label the boxes clearly for each of the serving times.

Set aside a specific time each week to fill all of the patient's medication boxes in one go. Schedule this task in your weekly plan so it's part of your regular routine and happens at a predictable time, such as every Sunday evening.

1. Fill all seven compartments of one box before filling the next box. For example, fill the morning serving, then the noon serving. Refer to the patient's medication schedule as you fill the compartments to prevent mistakes.

2. Ask someone to double-check your work to ensure correctness. The number of medications and their multiple serving times increases the likelihood of mistakes, and another pair of eyes helps catch many of these mistakes. Also, having someone who is familiar with the patient's medication regimen will be helpful in case you are unable to perform this task for any reason.

3. At the same time that you fill the boxes, review your medication inventory and make a list of what you will need for the following week. Order refills as necessary.

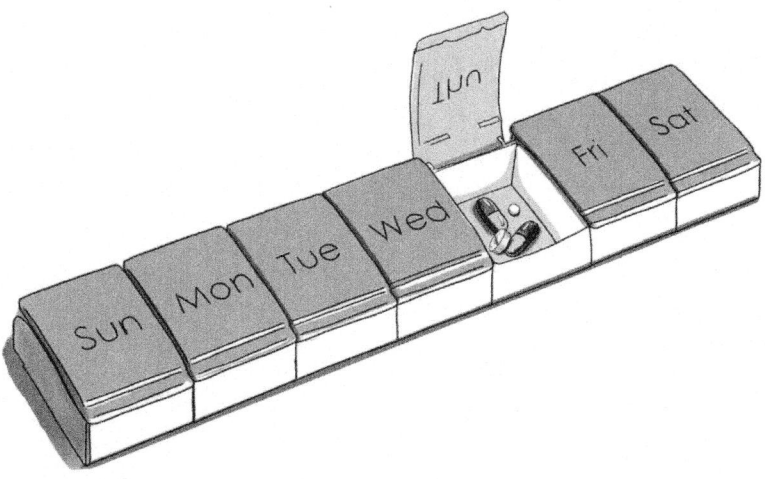

Figure 14.2 Medication box

Day-to-Day Management of Medications

- Once you have filled the medication boxes for each serving time, the meds are all in one place, ready to be administered at the appropriate times.

- If you try to serve a medication twice by mistake, you will immediately notice that the specific compartment is empty, signaling that the medication has been administered already.

- If you forget to administer one serving, you will notice this mistake the next time you inspect the medication box.

- Should you forget one serving, administer that serving as soon as you realize it. However, if you are close to the next serving time, do not serve the missed dose. When in doubt, consult your doctor.

You may want to use an app on your smartphone or other mobile device to remind you when it is time for the next serving of medication. As always, the best technique is to have medication times scheduled in the patient's daily routine.

15 | INCONTINENCE

Incontinence is the involuntary discharge of urine, stool, or both. It can be minor, involving only a few drops of urine or a small amount of stool, or it can be major, with a complete uncontrolled discharge.

Incontinence is a prominent feature of dementia, generally happening during the late stage, and sometimes as early as the middle stage. When it first happens, it's a shocking experience for both the patient and their caregiver. Although incontinence is something that will happen sooner or later, it often makes its debut when it's least expected, and most inconvenient.

Incontinence can remain unnoticed by family members and caregivers for a long time. It is a source of significant embarrassment for patients, who will do everything possible to hide it from others.

In the beginning, incontinence is sporadic, but slowly it turns into an everyday affair. The best you can do is to prepare for it and learn how to handle it before it arrives on the scene. From then on, it will be a constant companion for the rest of the journey.

Why It Happens

While incontinence can happen at any age, it is more common in older people. It is usually the result of weakness of the muscles that control urine and stool discharge. Women sometimes develop minor urinary incontinence that results in occasional discharge of small amounts of urine when they cough, sneeze, or laugh. Men may develop minor urinary incontinence due to prostate problems. Major incontinence, in contrast, is usually due to underlying diseases and medication side effects.

Incontinence and Dementia

> *My mom wakes up in the morning and sits at the edge of her bed. She does not respond to our cues to get up and go to the bathroom. This continues until she wets her pants.*

In dementia, incontinence has its roots in the progressive destruction of brain cells. As brain processing capacity is increasingly impaired, the chain of events from sensing the need to go to the bathroom, to understanding that sensation, to neuromuscular activation to get up and find one's way to the bathroom is interrupted, impairing the patient's ability to handle this most routine of daily and personal activities. The problem is compounded by a number of related issues:

- The patient may realize the urge to use the bathroom too late.

- After realizing the need to go, the patient's reaction may be slow and further hindered by joint stiffness and arthritis pain.

- The patient may refuse to accept help. They may be embarrassed and prefer to use the bathroom alone. They might be trying to hide their incontinence from others.

- The patient may not be able to express that they need to use the bathroom to get the assistance they need from their caregiver. They may have difficulty understanding when a caregiver asks if they need to go or reminds them that it is time to go.

- The patient may not be able to find the bathroom. They may be confused about its location and may not remember how to use it. They might confuse the flowerpot or the garbage bin for a toilet.

- The patient may reach the bathroom and then be confused as to what to do next. They may not remember how to pull their pants down and sit on the toilet.

Contributing Factors

Other factors contributing to incontinence may be grouped into three broad categories:

- Underlying diseases and conditions
- Side effects of drugs or other substances
- Environmental factors.

Underlying Conditions

- Urinary tract infection and an enlarged prostate both increase the risks of developing urinary incontinence.

- Constipation makes it more difficult to hold urine in or to empty one's bladder completely. Constipation may also result in soft stool leaking past the solid blockage in the large intestine, leading to fecal incontinence.

- Physical and movement disorders such as arthritis or joint pain may make it difficult to get to the bathroom in time.

- Stroke, type 2 diabetes, Parkinson's and other diseases that affect muscle control may also affect the muscles responsible for control of urine and stool discharge.

Medication Side Effects

- Muscle relaxants, such as those prescribed for sleep or anxiety, also affect muscles responsible for control of urine and stool discharge.

- Diuretic drugs, sometimes prescribed to lower blood pressure or for other medical reasons, require more frequent visits to the bathroom.

- Carbonated drinks, beer, tea, and coffee tend to increase urine volume, thereby increasing the risk of urinary incontinence.

Environmental Factors

- A patient waking up in the middle of the night to go to the bathroom may be confused about time and place, and may not be able to find the bathroom in time.

- Obstruction of the path to the bathroom by clutter, furniture, flower pots, and children's toys will not only create a fall hazard, but will also delay the patient's access to the bathroom.

- Certain types of clothing may prove too cumbersome for the patient to remove in time to use the toilet. Pants with an elastic waistband are easier to remove than those with belts and zippers.

When to See a Doctor

Incontinence affects all dementia patients sooner or later. Yet, patients are often reluctant to discuss it with their doctor. There are no drug-based interventions to stop incontinence generally. However, if the incontinence is due to some underlying condition, such as urinary tract infection or constipation, your doctor may be able to prescribe antibiotics or other interventions as necessary.

PREPARING FOR INCONTINENCE

Little by little, he couldn't find the bathroom anymore.

Long before the first bout of incontinence, you can begin to set the stage to delay its onset or reduce its effects. Once incontinence does arrive on the scene, these same precautions now baked into the patient's daily routine can help reduce the burden of incontinence for everyone involved.

Structure Routines to Improve Incontinence

- Encourage the patient to go to the bathroom every hour. Make bathroom visits a regularly scheduled activity in the patient's daily routine.

- Make a mental note of the patient's movements, behavior, and utterances when they need to use the bathroom. Then watch for those clues to detect when it is time to lead the patient to the bathroom.

- Have the patient wear loose-fitting clothes that are easy to remove during bathroom visits. Pants with an elastic band are easier to manage than those with a belt or a zipper.

- The patient may need to be alone when using the bathroom. If so, leave the bathroom but stay in the vicinity to prevent any problems.

- Make sure the patient sits on the toilet long enough to relieve themselves completely. Check the toilet afterwards to see if the task has been completed, and note the color and consistency as appropriate. Record it in the daily log for future reference.

Make It Easy to Find and Use the Bathroom

- Remove all clutter, extra furniture, children's toys, and other obstructions from the path to the bathroom to ensure easy access and to prevent falls.

- Remove any trash bins and flowerpots from the path to the bathroom so they are not mistaken for the toilet.

- If the path to the bathroom is carpeted, cover it with inexpensive, plain carpet. If this carpet is soiled, it will be much easier to clean than the rug or carpet underneath.

- Remove or cover carpets and rugs that have patterns on them. The patient may misperceive the patterns as flowers or other obstructions, and may get confused navigating them.

- Use contrasting color tape to clearly mark the path to the bathroom. This will make it easier for the patient to find the bathroom in dimmer lighting, at night, or when confused.

- The hallway and the path to the bathroom should be properly lit at all times. You can equip these areas with motion sensors to turn on the lights automatically when someone walks by.

- Mark the bathroom door with a sign identifying its purpose. Use a sign with a picture of a toilet and/or the word "Toilet" written on it. Place the sign at the patient's eye level, where they are sure to see it.

- White toilet seats, white tiles, and white walls may make it hard for the patient to see the toilet clearly. Choose a dark color toilet seat, or use washable colored adhesives to make the toilet seat stand out.

- Make the bathroom easy to use. Install a higher toilet seat, toilet safety rails, and grab bars to make it easier for the patient to sit down and get up.

- Put a medical commode or a bathroom wheelchair in the patient's bedroom for quicker access at night.

HOW TO HANDLE INCONTINENCE

We were at the grocery store when I heard my wife mumble "No, no, no!" as her pants started to get wet. She was standing in the middle of the aisle. I moved closer and stood next to her for support and whispered, "Don't worry. It's okay." I waited until she had finished, then said, "Let's go." I didn't say anything else, and neither did she. We just walked out of the store, hand in hand.

It's hard to imagine the anxiety that someone may feel as they experience incontinence developing for the first time and realize that they are gradually losing control over the most fundamental aspects of their existence. They may get depressed, cry every time it happens, and be deeply embarrassed by it. They may try to help the problem by visiting the bathroom repeatedly, especially when they're about to leave home to go somewhere.

Be Supportive

- Treat the patient with love and respect, and do not show any sign of anxiety or embarrassment. Communicate in ways that lighten the mood. Instead of saying, "You wet your pants again!" say, "Something spilled on your pants?"

- Your approach should be matter-of-fact and natural so the patient does not feel guilty or embarrassed.

- Do not infantilize the patient. Avoid words and phrases that one might use to encourage children to go to the bathroom to avoid accidents.

Helping the Patient to the Bathroom

My mother sits in her chair for long hours, even when her diaper is soiled. She does not let us take her to the bathroom or change her.

Well into the course of dementia progression, the patient will likely remain reluctant to allow someone to help them in this most private of tasks. When trying to help the patient, do not give them the impression that you want to do something against their will. Instead, find ways around cognitive obstacles and hang-ups. Go with the flow, rather than fight it.

1. Approach the patient from the front so they can see you and have time to process what is happening.

2. Kneel next to the patient's chair.

3. Bring your hand toward the patient as though you are asking them to put their hand in yours. Wait until they comply with your request.

4. With hands locked in a gentle handshake position, greet the patient as you would if you hadn't seen them in weeks. Tell them that you are very happy to see them.

5. Shift your hand from a handshake hold to an arm wrestling hold. With this hold, you can more comfortably help the patient to get up and walk.

6. Make a gesture of getting up and help the patient to get up as well.

7. Don't talk about the bathroom or any soiled clothes.

8. Walk slowly to the bathroom.

9. Once in the bathroom, lower the patient's pants with the help of their own hand still being held in yours so the patient feels that they are the one doing it.

10. Relax and take your time. Do not rush things so the patient does not feel that you are forcing them into something they don't want to do.

11. Stay friendly and inject some humor into the process. Sing the tunes the patient loves and continue speaking to them in a nice and relaxed manner. Do not talk about the toilet affair.

Cleaning the Patient Afterwards

- If the patient is unable to clean themselves after using the bathroom, help them in a respectful way. Ask for their permission to help them. Treat them as you would if they were healthy.

- Approach the task gently so the patient feels comfortable allowing you to clean them. Otherwise, they may insist on doing it themselves and end up making a mess. Unable to clean properly, they may soil their clothes or their genital area, setting the stage for urinary tract or other infection.

- While you are cleaning the patient, they may grab your hand and prevent you from completing the task. If so, give them a small object, like a soft ball or a towel, to hold for you.

Stay Calm in the Middle of Mayhem

After helping my dad to the toilet, I stepped out briefly to check my email. A minute or two later, I noticed him going from room to room, naked from the waist down and bewildered, his hands cupped together full of feces. As I scrambled to contain the situation, my sister descended upon us, screaming and cursing. Here I was in the middle, trying to help Dad to the bathroom as he was trying to hand his payload over to me, and my sister screaming into my ear at the top of her lungs, all the way to the bathroom and beyond.

Sometimes behaviors associated with bathroom and incontinence may seem bizarre at first. The patient may put their hands in their pants and then wipe their soiled hands on the wall to clean them. Or, they may manage to remove their pants and underwear, but then forgetting what to do next, may defecate in their own hands. They might mistake another room for the toilet, lift the corner of the rug like a toilet seat cover, do their business on the floor, and then put the rug back down over it.

As with everything else in dementia, you have to deal with such behaviors in a calm and collected way. The patient is already confused. Any frustration, agitation, or cursing on your part will only make things worse. Instead, try to reassure the patient with kindness so they feel comfortable allowing you to help them. You must be prepared to give up whatever you are doing, calmly take the patient's hand and, without a lot of talking, walk them to the bathroom.

In general, the caregiver should accompany the patient into the bathroom. If the patient does not allow you to remain in the bathroom, stay close and vigilant so you can intervene if they forget what to do or start to make a mess. Above all, intervene in a calm and friendly manner. Although the patient may not be comfortable with your presence initially, if your help comes tactfully and with due respect for their privacy, they will slowly begin to trust you to help them.

INCONTINENCE HYGIENE

Incontinence increases the risks of medical complications, including urinary tract infection (UTI), and UTI in turn increases the frequency and severity of incontinence. UTI is also a major health hazard as it can lead to more serious, even life-threatening, consequences. When facing incontinence, preventing UTI is a primary concern.

Prevent Rashes and Infections

- Ensure proper hygiene. Wash and clean the patient at least twice each day: in the morning after waking up, and at night before going to bed.

- In addition to washing as part of a regular hygiene routine, wash and clean the patient thoroughly after each bout of fecal incontinence.

- Pat dry the patient well after each wash to prevent skin damage, rashes, and burns. Do not rub a towel on the patient's skin to dry, as it may cause the fragile skin to break.

- Use baby cream or other gentle moisturizer on the washed areas to prevent the skin from getting dry and itchy.

- Apply a generous amount of zinc oxide cream to the skin that came into contact with stool or urine to treat or prevent skin irritations. If the skin is very dry, you can use zinc oxide ointment instead, which contains more oil for better protection against moisture loss.

- Damaged skin is prone to infection. Inspect the patient's body for any signs of burns, irritation, scratches, insect bites, or other skin injuries. Do this regularly, and especially after each wash.

- Examine the patient's clothes regularly and change any wet or dirty clothes right away. Wash any soiled clothes as soon as possible, and sun-dry the clothes if possible.

Use a Variety of Pads for Protection

Incontinence supplies are available in both disposable and washable/reusable types and come in a variety of absorbency levels.

- Line the patient's underwear with absorbent incontinence pads to help prevent urine from seeping through to the patient's underwear, pants, and the furniture.

- Incontinence pads can keep underwear from getting soiled, if the pads are checked often. Checking the pads every thirty minutes, and changing them even if slightly wet, reduces the need to change the rest of the patient's underwear and pants. It also helps prevent UTI.

- For heavier or more frequent incontinence, use incontinence shorts. These shorts have good absorption, making them suitable for brief outings, such as a visit to the doctor.

- Incontinence shorts are a good option during the day, especially if the patient still has relatively good cognition. These shorts look and feel more like regular underwear, making it more likely that the patient will agree to wear them.

- For longer periods of time, such as overnight, use adult diapers.

- Use underpads to protect furniture and bed sheets against accidents. Underpads come in a variety of sizes and are available in two types: disposable and washable. The washable type has thick cotton lining, which makes it more suitable for situations where the patient's skin comes into direct contact with the underpad.

When Going Out

Preventing UTI remains a priority when you go out. In the event of an incontinence episode, the cleaning, washing, drying, and changing of the patient must be done properly, regardless of whether you are at home or outside.

Before going out, assess the risks and plan ahead. Think through the steps needed to clean and change the patient should an incontinence episode arise. What do you need to accomplish the task properly? Is there a place where you can do that safely and with reasonable privacy? Can you handle cleaning and dressing the patient alone, with all the patience and stamina that it requires? Will the patient cooperate with you or will it end in agitation and anger?

If you are not confident that you can manage all of the above, it may be better to forgo the outing or get extra help if you do need to leave home. In any event, make sure you have all the necessary supplies packed and ready in case you ever need to leave in a hurry.

- Use a carry-on bag and pack everything you need to handle an incontinence episode when you are away from home.

- Pack a complete change of clothes including pants and socks, incontinence pads and shorts, latex gloves, plastic bags to store soiled clothes, paper towels, wipes, soap and water, hand sanitizer, and other accessories necessary for a thorough job.

- Replenish the supplies after each outing. Keep the carry-on bag well stocked so it's always ready to go.

HYDRATION AND INCONTINENCE

My father is in the late stage of Alzheimer's disease. He urinates only once every 24 hours.

It's easy to lose sight of adequate hydration when you're trying to manage incontinence. However, dehydration is a real threat and can lead to UTI and constipation, two of the most important concerns relating to incontinence. Not only do UTI and constipation increase the risks of incontinence, they are also major risk factors for a variety of other medical and health complications.

- An individual needs about eight glasses of fluids daily to prevent dehydration. Make sure the patient's daily schedule includes adequate servings of fluids.

- Do not reduce the patient's fluid intake in the hopes of preventing incontinence. Monitor the patient's daily log to make sure you're not inadvertently curbing their fluid intake.

- Watch for infrequent urination, or abnormally little output, as they may be signs of dehydration. In men, urination issues may also be a result of an enlarged prostate.

- Manage the patient's hydration schedule so you won't have to serve them fluids within two hours prior to their bedtime.

- Take the patient to the bathroom before bedtime, and make sure they empty their bladder completely.

INCONTINENCE OVERNIGHT

Incontinence is especially stressful at night, as it disturbs the patient's and the caregiver's sleep. You can make the experience less stressful by planning ahead to make the process of changing sheets, clothes, and underpads streamlined and easier.

Plan Ahead

With the right precautions in place, nighttime incontinence episodes are usually handled quickly, often by simply changing the patient's pajamas and underpads.

- Cover the patient's mattress with a waterproof mattress cover.

- For added protection, put a large underpad under the bed sheet, and another one over the bed sheet.

- When putting the patient to bed, roll up the back of their pajama top above their hips so if the underpad gets wet, their pajama top remains dry.

- Keep all the necessary supplies in the patient's bedroom for easy access. You'll need spare pajamas, underpads, sheets, a wastebasket, latex gloves, baby wipes, and paper towels.

- In case of fecal incontinence, wear two latex gloves on each hand. After the initial wiping, discard the outer gloves to prevent contaminating clean items. With the outer gloves discarded, you still have a pair of clean gloves on to complete the cleaning process.

Use Appropriate Sleepwear

My dad is incontinent. During the day, my mom takes him to the bathroom at regular intervals. At night, he wears diapers and pajamas to bed, but we find him naked and totally wet in the morning.

Nighttime can be especially confusing for the patient. They may wake up feeling the need to go to the bathroom and may even manage to undress in time, only to forget what to do next. Or, they may think that they are already in the bathroom and relieve themselves in bed.

- Early on, convenient sleepwear such as loose-fitting T-shirt and pull-up pants can help simplify bathroom visits at night. Over time, additional measures such as incontinence pads and shorts, or adult diapers will become necessary.

- Eventually, simple pajamas or pull-up pants may become impractical because the patient may keep removing them. If so, have the patient wear a one-piece sleepwear, or union suit, so they cannot undress easily at night.

Watch for Signs of Discomfort

My father wears a one-piece jump-suit to bed, but somehow still manages to pull out his diaper in the middle of the night.

Wearing a diaper for long hours can get uncomfortable. The patient may feel hot in the diaper, or may have skin rash or other irritation. Other potential causes of discomfort include constipation, urinary tract infection, or enlarged prostate.

Approach behavioral issues by trying to discover and eliminate the root causes of the problem.

- Does the diaper get hot at night?

- Does the patient's skin show signs of irritation, rash, scratches, or insect bites?

- Is the patient constipated? The associated feeling that they need to go to the bathroom can make the patient try to undress.

- Does the patient have urinary tract infection? UTI is associated with burning sensation and frequent urination.

- Does the patient suffer from an enlarged prostate? An enlarged prostate does not allow the bladder to empty completely, leaving the patient with a persistent feeling that they need to go to the bathroom.

Behavioral issues are often clues to underlying discomfort. Approach them as opportunities to identify and resolve the pain that the patient may be suffering in silence. Stay vigilant to notice them at first sign, and spring into action to relieve the patient's discomfort quickly and effectively.

CATHETERS AND LATE-STAGE INCONTINENCE

In late stage dementia, when the patient is bedridden, it might be tempting to use a catheter instead of a diaper to manage urinary incontinence. This is not a decision to be taken lightly.

Diapers provide better visibility and control. Urinary catheters don't provide a lot of visibility into what is going on, which may give you a false sense of security. Furthermore, catheters are generally not intended for long-term use, except in special circumstances.

Catheters are prone to causing urinary tract infection, mainly due to contamination during the insertion and removal of the catheter. As a result, they have similar infection risks for men and women. External urinary catheters, such as condom catheters, tend to pose a lower risk of infection compared to regular catheters, and with much less discomfort.

16 | Critical Health Issues

Dementia is accompanied by a number of common and recurring health conditions, such as urinary tract infections, aspiration pneumonia, and bedsores. These conditions can develop suddenly and, if left untreated, can escalate to serious, even life-threatening, levels rapidly.

Caring for a loved one with dementia is an exercise in monitoring and prevention. You must stay continuously on the lookout for warning signs of problems brewing and act quickly to resolve any issues before they grow into crises that can upend your entire caregiving enterprise.

URINARY TRACT INFECTION

The urinary tract or the urinary system is a group of organs that work together to extract waste products from the blood stream, and expel them from the body in the form of urine. The system includes two kidneys that remove wastes from the blood stream, a tube from each kidney to the bladder where urine is collected, and the urethra through which the bladder empties.

How Do Urinary Tract Infections Start?

Under normal conditions, the urinary system and the urine that it produces are free from bacteria and other infectious agents. Urinary tract infections (UTI) are caused when external agents such as bacteria, fungi, and viruses enter the urinary tract. Infection usually starts at the mouth of the urethra and, if left untreated, gradually spreads upstream to other parts of the urinary system.

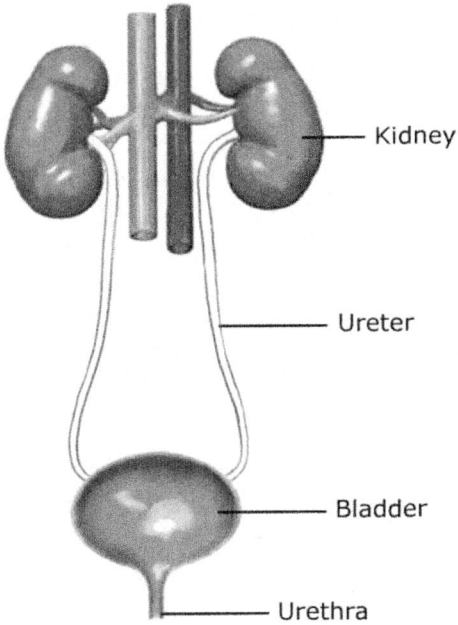

Kidney

Ureter

Bladder

Urethra

Figure 16.1 The urinary system.
When healthy, it is free from bacteria and other agents.

UTI in Dementia

UTI is a common feature of dementia, especially during the middle and late stages. Patients' weakened immune system, incontinence, and inadequate hygiene contribute to making UTI a constant challenge.

- Due to anatomical differences between men and women, the internal urinary system in women is more accessible to bacteria and other infectious agents entering through the urethra. This is why women are advised to wipe front to back after going to the bathroom, to reduce the risk of developing UTI.

- As muscles of the bladder weaken with age, it becomes harder to empty the bladder completely. A semi-empty bladder, coupled with incontinence, can lead to more frequent incidence of UTI.

- Contact with wet and soiled pads and diapers makes it easier for bacteria to enter the urethra. Promptly replace pads when they get soiled. Visit the bathroom regularly to minimize the risk of soiled underwear and wash the patient frequently.

- Over time, the patient grows less and less able to perform personal hygiene routines properly. They may perform tasks incorrectly, may not get a complete wash as often, and may not be able to do a thorough cleaning due to balance and other issues.

Symptoms of UTI

Symptoms of UTI vary from person to person. If the infection is in the lower urinary system, the symptoms are milder than if the infection has spread to the upper part.

A UTI that hasn't spread beyond the bladder is considered the mild type. The most common symptoms of lower UTI are:

- Burning sensation during urination

- Frequent urination in small amounts

- Pain and pressure in the back and lower abdomen

- Dark, cloudy, or bloody urine, sometimes with an unusual odor

- Fatigue or shivering

- Mild fever up to 100.4 Fahrenheit (38 Celsius).

If the infection spreads beyond the bladder, the infection is more severe and will be harder to treat. In addition to the above symptoms, upper UTI may involve:

- Nausea and pain in the sides

- Severe chills and high fever around 102.2 to 104°F (39 to 40°C).

Symptoms in Patients With Dementia

In patients with dementia, UTI may present with or without fever and other symptoms typical of this condition. However, UTI is often accompanied with behavioral changes that can be clues to something going on behind the scenes.

- Patients with dementia may not exhibit many of the symptoms of UTI. Additionally, they are often unable to communicate their pain and discomfort.

- UTI in patients with dementia may cause behavioral changes such as confusion, anxiety, restlessness, aggression, lethargy, and becoming withdrawn. Be on the lookout for behavioral changes as signs of problems brewing in the background.

- Among the warning signs of possible UTI is a sudden loss of abilities such as a sudden loss of balance, or a sudden inability to walk or eat on their own.

- Stay vigilant for the subtle signs of a UTI developing. UTIs should be treated promptly. Keep in mind that any infection can speed up the progression of dementia or intensify its symptoms.

In later stages of dementia, when the patient is unable to communicate their discomfort, it is especially important to watch for subtle signs of UTI. Closed eyes during the day, tendency to sleep more than usual, lethargy, and increased bouts of incontinence are indications that something is wrong. At the first sign of a possible UTI, spring into action to test for and contain it right away.

Testing for UTI

To diagnose a UTI, your doctor will usually rely on a urine test, or urinalysis. You can perform a test at home using disposable urine test strips that you can buy over the counter. Or you can collect a urine sample and have it tested at a lab. Naturally, the home test is not as accurate as a test performed at a lab.

A home test only detects if UTI is present. A lab, however, can grow a urine culture to determine the specific type of bacteria present, and the right antibiotic to target the bacteria. It usually takes two to three days for the results of a urine culture to be ready.

- Perform a urine culture every time UTI is suspected. This is to ensure that you are targeting the right bacteria with the right antibiotics, and not losing precious time shooting in the dark.

Obtaining a Urine Sample

Getting a urine sample is not easy. In the early stages of dementia, the patient may not cooperate, and in the middle and late stages, incontinence will make it hard to obtain a urine sample. Still, with a little planning and a lot of care, you can obtain a viable urine sample even during the middle and late stages of dementia progression.

1. Use a disposable bowl to collect the urine sample.

2. Wash and dry the bowl to remove any contaminant.

3. Place the bowl inside the toilet bowl so it floats on the water. Take care to not contaminate the inside of the bowl in the process.

4. The next time you take the patient to the bathroom, you may get a urine sample collected in the disposable bowl.

5. Remove the disposable bowl from the toilet and place it on a newspaper or paper towel to dry the bottom of the bowl.

6. Transfer the sample from the disposable bowl to the lab container, taking care to not contaminate the sample.

This approach works well; however, collecting discharged urine is prone to contamination, especially for female patients. To reduce the risk of contamination, disinfect the genital area with sterile gauze and ladies disinfectant gel before taking a urine sample. The alternative is to use a catheter to collect a sample directly from the bladder. A trained nurse should perform this operation.

Treating UTI

If the result of the urine test is positive, your doctor will usually prescribe an oral antibiotic. With prompt action, UTI can usually be treated with a single course of oral antibiotics. However, if the infection is not treated properly, it may spread to the bladder and onward to the kidneys, resulting in life-threatening complications.

- Make sure that the patient takes the antibiotics all the way through the period prescribed by their doctor. Do not stop the meds after partial recovery.

- At the first sign of UTI and through the course of treatment, increase the patient's fluid intake to increase urine volume and help flush out the bacteria.

- Do not medicate the patient on your own, and do not administer antibiotics without a doctor's prescription. Taking antibiotics on your own may create resistance in the bacteria, so when you really need the antibiotics, they may no longer work.

Preventing UTI

Urinary tract infections make life more difficult for the patient and their caregiver. More than that, frequent UTI and the associated antibiotic use increase the risk that someday you may come across a type of bacteria that is resistant to treatment. It is therefore imperative to reduce the frequency of UTIs through proper care and prevention.

Drink Plenty of Fluids

- An individual with normal body weight and average level of activity requires six to eight glasses of water daily to stay properly hydrated. Dehydration is one of the causes of UTI and one of the easiest to prevent.

- Make sure that the patient does not hold in their urine for long periods of time. Remind them to go to the bathroom or take them if they are unable to go on their own. Have them visit the bathroom at specific intervals, such as every hour.

Clean Properly

- Replace incontinence pads and diapers promptly if wet.

- If the patient is still managing their hygiene alone, make sure they are doing it correctly. Sooner or later, they will need more help with cleaning and washing.

- Wash the patient carefully at least twice a day, once when they wake up, and again when they go to bed at night. In case of a bowel movement in their shorts or diapers, wash them again thoroughly.

- Warm and humid areas are ideal environments for bacteria and fungi to grow. Use a blow drier to dry the washed area after you have wiped it with a towel.

- For female patients, use sterile gauze and ladies disinfectant gel, and disinfect from the front to the back. Do not repeat the front-to-back motion with the same gauze, or you run the risk of spreading germs back to the front.

Make Urine More Acidic

- Most bacteria do not grow in acidic environments. Make urine more acidic by including plenty of vitamin C in the patient's diet. You can use vitamin C pills or cranberry pills, which are available as over-the-counter dietary supplements at your local pharmacy.

- Orange juice, cranberry juice, and blueberries are excellent sources of vitamin C. Serve fruit juices freshly squeezed, rather than processed, as the processed variety usually contains a lot of added sugar.

- Parsley is also rich in vitamin C. Include it fresh in the patient's diet. If the patient has trouble chewing, mince the parsley with a knife and serve it on their soup or other food.

Maintenance Antibiotics

- Your doctor may prescribe a low-dose antibiotic to be taken daily to prevent UTI. However, antibiotics may also kill the good bacteria that are necessary for digestive health. This may result in diarrhea, frequent bowel movements, or runny stool. If so, your doctor may stop the low-dose antibiotics altogether.

- Use probiotic dairy products or food supplements to replenish the good bacteria that are lost as a result of taking antibiotics. You may also make your own probiotic yogurt by using kefir starter grains.

CONSTIPATION

Constipation is a recurring problem in dementia, and tends to get worse over time. A number of factors contribute to constipation in dementia, including reduction in mobility with advancing dementia, drinking less water to reduce incontinence, eating less fruits and vegetables due to chewing difficulties, and generally turning to diets that contain less fiber, such as pudding and ice cream. Consequently, all the necessary ingredients are in place for recurrent constipation.

Constipation is a serious health issue and can lead to other complications, such as urinary blockage, fecal incontinence, and subsequent UTI due to possible contamination. As a result, it remains one of the primary areas of concern for caregivers throughout the course of dementia progression.

Preventing Constipation

If the patient does not have a bowel movement three days in a row, they are considered constipated. Aim for a bowel movement at least every other day, or three times per week, in order to prevent constipation.

- Include physical activity and stretches in the patient's daily routine. Even mild exercise, such as walking and simple gardening, can help prevent constipation.

- Keep the patient on a healthy diet that includes vegetables, fresh fruits, foods rich in dietary fiber like peas and beans, and nuts like almonds and walnuts.

- If a diet high in fiber-rich foods is not enough to prevent constipation, you can use dietary fiber as a supplement.

- Keep the patient properly hydrated. Reduce the consumption of coffee, tea, soft drinks, and alcohol, and substitute water instead.

Treating Constipation

My mother hasn't had a bowel movement in five days. I have given her different forms of common laxatives, but nothing has worked so far. At this point we're starting to think an enema might be the only option.

Treat constipation promptly before it becomes a chronic problem. Like most other problems in dementia, constipation is harder to resolve the longer it goes untreated.

- If the patient does not have a bowel movement in two consecutive days, start home remedies right away.

- Soaked dried prunes and peaches are rich in fiber and are good remedies for constipation. Prune juice works well, too.

- Milk of magnesia, available over the counter, or a tablespoon of olive oil at bedtime may solve the problem.

- Do not use laxatives without consulting with your doctor. Do not let laxatives become a regular part of your care routine, in lieu of proper diet, hydration, and physical activity.

- Do not use suppositories or resort to enemas without prior consultation with your doctor, and even then, only sparingly. Due to patients' fragile condition, especially in the late stage of dementia, such interventions can lead to other complications.

Staying Regular

- Maintain a regular daily schedule to ensure that the patient's needs are being met, from physical activity and exercise to nutrition, hydration, and adequate fiber intake. A consistent daily schedule is critical in keeping bowel movements regular.

- The best time for a bowel movement is early in the morning upon waking up. Organize the patient's daily and weekly schedule, including meals, snacks, fluids, activity and exercise, to facilitate regular timing of bowel movement on most days.

- Record bowel movements, including quantity and quality, in the patient's daily activity log. Monitor the daily log to keep track of the patient's condition over days and weeks, and identify potential issues before they develop into crises.

Adopt a Modified Squat Posture

To facilitate bowel movement, adopt a more natural posture:

- Once the patient is sitting on the toilet, put a small pedestal under their feet to bring their knees up and closer to their abdomen. This is a more natural posture for bowel movement than sitting up on a toilet seat.

- Lean the patient slightly forward to better approximate the natural squatting posture.

Always Check Afterwards

Do not rely on the patient's self-report about the success of their bathroom visits. Make a point of verifying it yourself, every time. Proper verification not only helps catch common issues such as constipation and dehydration early on, it also helps alert you to other potentially serious medical conditions, such as intestinal blockage or urinary tract obstruction.

The plane had just taken off when my husband needed to use the restroom. As the flight attendants walked the aisles tending to other passengers, I stood guard at the bathroom door with my husband inside. A few minutes later, we made our way back to our seats, and right away he had to go to the bathroom again. An hour into the flight, cabin lights had been switched off and the other passengers had settled in for the long flight. And we were still shuffling back and forth between our seats and the restroom.

A couple hours into the flight, the head flight attendant made an announcement over the intercom: there was a passenger with urinary tract obstruction who needed medical attention. Was there a doctor on the plane? The back of the plane became a makeshift emergency room. I stood outside as my husband screamed over the sound of the engines. Eventually, the doctor came out, dripping with sweat. He said my husband hadn't urinated in four days. He had an enlarged prostate, which had made it impossible to insert a catheter. He needed emergency medical attention.

The cabin lights came on, and the pilot made an announcement: there was a medical emergency on board and we were diverting to a nearby airport. On the ground, emergency crews were standing by, and soon we were on our way, with sirens blaring, to the hospital. On the way, my husband kept staring at me with angry eyes, like he was blaming me for what had happened. And I kept hearing the doctor's voice echo in the howling sirens: "How could you not know that you have to check up on him in the bathroom every time?"

Pneumonia

It's 2am. My husband is up again. I can hear his father's breathing from the other room. His aspiration pneumonia is bad this time. I hear the sound of the electric suction device. 3am, the sound of suction wakes me up again. I check on the baby. She's still asleep. 4am, my husband is beside himself. Power is out and neither the suction device, nor the oxygen machine work. 4:30, power is back on. Suction again. 5am, I get up to feed the baby. I see my mother in law in the other room tending to her husband. 6am, the baby is crying again. My husband is fast asleep, exhausted. I pick up the baby and hurry to suction his dad. 7am, time to tend to his bedsores. More suction.

Pneumonia is an infection of the lungs, where the air sacs in one or both lungs are inflamed and fill with fluid, making breathing difficult. It is a serious condition and requires immediate medical attention.

Who Is at Risk?

Pneumonia can happen to anyone, but people over 65, children younger than two years old, and people with underlying conditions are at a higher risk. Patients in the late stage of dementia are especially at risk, due to impaired swallowing and reduced immune system function.

Symptoms of Pneumonia

Symptoms of pneumonia vary from mild to severe, but in all cases should be taken very seriously. This is especially true for the elderly, those with underlying health conditions, and dementia patients.
Watch for:

- Coughing, especially when accompanied by phlegm that is yellow, green, or brown in color, or with visible blood

- Difficulty breathing, with short, shallow breaths

- Fever, usually above 102°F (39°C)

- Heart rate that is faster than usual

- Chills accompanied by sweating

- Decreased blood oxygen, as measured on a home pulse oximeter.

Symptoms in Patients With Dementia

Dementia patients don't always exhibit obvious symptoms of an infection, such as a fever. You'll have to be on the lookout for more subtle signs, such as changes in behavior or breathing difficulties, in order to catch it early on.

- Even during severe infections, dementia patients may not develop much of a fever.

- Infections, including pneumonia, typically cause behavioral changes such as confusion, anxiety, lethargy, and other changes in awareness and mood.

Treatment

See your doctor immediately if you suspect pneumonia. Your doctor will examine the patient and listen to their lungs. They may order imaging studies, blood tests, or other lab work to determine the cause of the infection, and the type of antibiotics needed to treat it.

If diagnosed early, pneumonia may be treated in seven to ten days with oral antibiotics. In more severe cases, the patient may need to be hospitalized for intravenous (IV) antibiotics and closer monitoring.

Aspiration Pneumonia

Pneumonia is an ever-present danger over the course of dementia progression. Swallowing problems during the late stage, and sometimes in the middle stage, make meal times dangerous and stressful.

- Aspiration refers to food or liquids entering the windpipe. It can also happen when saliva or stomach acid (acid reflux) find their way into the windpipe.

- Aspiration is usually accompanied by severe coughing to expel the foreign material from the windpipe. With declining strength over time, patients gradually lose the ability to cough hard enough to accomplish this vital function.

- The accumulation of foreign matter inside the lungs causes an infection known as aspiration pneumonia. This is very common in dementia.

- When swallowing is impaired, aspiration may occur without coughing or other indications. This is referred to as silent aspiration.

Preventing Pneumonia

In the early stage of dementia, your doctor or speech therapist may be able to assess the patient's swallowing function and provide advice on how to reduce the risks of aspiration. With the development of swallowing problems, however, it is inevitable that some food or liquids will find their way into the patient's windpipe. Managing swallowing difficulties remains the key to preventing pneumonia, especially in the late stage of dementia progression.

- When feeding the patient, have them sit upright in a chair. Lean their head slightly forward to help close their windpipe during swallowing. Do not feed the patient while they are lying down.

- Feed the patient in a calm and quiet environment. Keep distractions to a minimum to reduce the chances of aspiration.

- Feed the patient in small bites. Do not feed them the next bite until you are sure that their mouth is empty.

- When necessary, use a blender or a food processor to puree the patient's meals to a consistency similar to that of thick yogurt. Add thickener to liquids as necessary to make them easier to swallow.

- Use mucolytic syrup to help discharge excess phlegm. Consult with your doctor for the type most appropriate for the patient.

- Perform lung physiotherapy at least twice a day to help dislodge phlegm from the patient's lungs and windpipe.

- Use a humidifier in the patient's bedroom to help make the air more comfortable for breathing, especially during cold months when the room air is dry.

- Take care to not contaminate the patient's mouth. Wash your hands frequently, especially before feeding the patient. If necessary, you can use hand sanitizer or other antiseptic gel.

- Pay attention to the health of the patient's teeth and gums. Tooth and gum infections increase the amount of harmful bacteria in the mouth, which can contaminate the lungs when saliva inevitably finds its way into the windpipe.

- Keep acid reflux under control. Acid reflux may cause small amounts of partially digested food and other stomach content to find their way back up to the mouth and into the windpipe and the lungs, causing aspiration pneumonia. Consult your doctor for help in controlling acid reflux.

BEDSORES AND PRESSURE ULCERS

If you apply pressure to a point on the skin, the pressure blocks blood flow through the capillaries at that point. If the pressure persists for a few hours, skin cells and the underlying tissue begin to die, creating a pressure ulcer. If the pressure continues still, the injury develops into an open sore, impacting muscle, bone, and other tissues at the affected area.

Pressure ulcers are often referred to as bedsores, since they usually develop as a result of prolonged confinement to bed.

Conditions such as diabetes, infections, hospitalization, incontinence, inadequate or improper nutrition, and reduced awareness as a result of dementia are some of the other factors contributing to the development of pressure ulcers.

Who Is at Risk?

While sitting or sleeping, a healthy individual shifts around and changes position naturally to avoid prolonged pressure on any point on their body. A person with a medical condition that limits their ability to change positions cannot relieve pressure adequately, and is therefore at risk of developing bedsores. Elderly people, those with limited mobility due to injury or illness, and people who spend most of their time in bed or in a chair are at risk.

Dementia and Bedsores

Dementia patients are at a greater risk of developing bedsores, especially during the late stage, when the patient is less mobile, has a weakened immune system, and cannot express their pain or discomfort. This makes bedsores more likely and their early detection more difficult. Early detection is critical, however, since bedsores tend to develop suddenly and, if left untreated, will progress rapidly. They are quite painful.

My dad keeps pulling his knees to his chest at night, which pulls his sheets off of him. To keep him from getting cold, I thought to strap his ankles to the bedpost at the foot of the bed. I used a soft fabric and was careful not to wrap his ankles too tightly. Still, within a couple of nights he developed sores on the front of both his ankles. I just can't bring myself to look him in the eyes anymore.

Prevention

Treating advanced bedsores is difficult and requires professional care. Advanced bedsores also take a long time to heal. Therefore, it is critical to prevent bedsores from developing in the first place. It takes vigilance to discover and treat bedsores right away, and to prevent them from advancing to more serious stages.

Daily Monitoring

- Monitor vulnerable areas on the patient's body in order to detect the first signs of potential trouble. Pay special attention to areas that are under pressure when sitting or lying down.

- Every morning after waking the patient up, inspect the areas of their body susceptible to pressure during sleep. A good time for this is during morning stretches while the patient is still in bed.

- Bathing time is an ideal opportunity to inspect the patient from head to toe for early signs of bedsores.

- To inspect an area, press it gently with your finger. If the skin is healthy, its color will turn white under your finger, and will return back to its natural color when you remove the pressure.

Patient Handling

- Do not leave the patient in one position for long periods.

- When in bed, turn the patient every two hours so no part of their body is subjected to continuous pressure for more than two hours at a time.

- Getting tangled up in bed sheets can put extra pressure on the skin. Prevent bed sheets from wrapping tightly around the patient's limbs overnight.

- Wet bedding creates more friction and increases the risk of skin damage. Change wet sheets and clothes right away.

- When moving the patient, take care to not stretch or pull on their skin. It takes a moment of carelessness to scratch, break, or tear fragile skin. During patient transfers, for example from bed to wheelchair, take extra care of the skin at the hips and buttocks.

Health and Hygiene

- The risks of developing advanced bedsores are higher if the patient is incontinent. A wound that comes into contact with urine or feces is in fertile grounds for infection.

- Staying hydrated helps keep skin healthy and fresh and reduces the risk of bedsores. Do not wait until the patient is thirsty to give them fluids. They may be unable to communicate that they are thirsty, or may not even be aware of it.

Use Pressure-Relief Equipment

- Invest in an alternating pressure mattress. These mattresses have air cells, such as tubes running laterally along the width of the mattress, or bladders arranged in a lattice, like an egg carton. An electric pump automatically inflates different groups of cells every few minutes, allowing others to deflate in turn. In this way, the pressure on the patient's body changes frequently without the need to move the patient.

- Use pressure relief seat cushions to reduce pressure on the patient's pelvis while sitting in a wheelchair. Some cushions have air- or water-filled pockets arranged like cells in an egg carton, giving a floating sensation.

- Alternatively, you may use a seat cushion made of high-density foam. These cushions sometimes have a U-shaped piece (around 4"x4") cut from the back end to reduce or eliminate pressure on the tailbone. If your cushion doesn't have this feature, you can cut away that part of the cushion yourself.

Vulnerable Areas

Any area of the body subject to sustained pressure is at risk of developing bedsores. However, skin that covers bony areas is especially at risk. Keep a close watch on the back of the head, ears, shoulders and shoulder blades, elbows, spine, tailbone, pelvis, hips, knees, ankles, heels, and toes.

- A quilt or a blanket, especially if tucked under the mattress at the foot of the bed, places pressure on the toes when the patient is sleeping on their back. To reduce the pressure, place a large pillow or cushion at the foot of the bed under the blanket, so the blanket is propped up like a tent and does not rest on the patient's toes.

- When the patient is lying on their back, the weight of their feet places sustained pressure on their heels. To relieve the pressure, place a thin pillow under the patient's legs close to the ankles, so the heels and ankles are propped off of the mattress.

- The hips carry a lot of weight and are at a constant risk of bedsores. When raising the back of the bed to put the patient in a more upright posture, proceed gently. The greater the angle, the greater the pressure on the buttocks, hips, and the tailbone.

- When sitting or lying in a bed with its back raised, the body's tendency to slide down exerts a shearing force on the patient's skin. To reduce the risk of damage to the skin, minimize the time spent in this position. Do not raise the back of the bed all the way up. If the bed has the capability, raise the knee area to reduce the downward slide.

- Some patients rub their thumb and index finger together constantly, wearing out their skin. Others may clench their fists tightly, digging their nails into the flesh of their palms. An effective solution for both is to place a soft ball or something similar in their hand to remove the pressure.

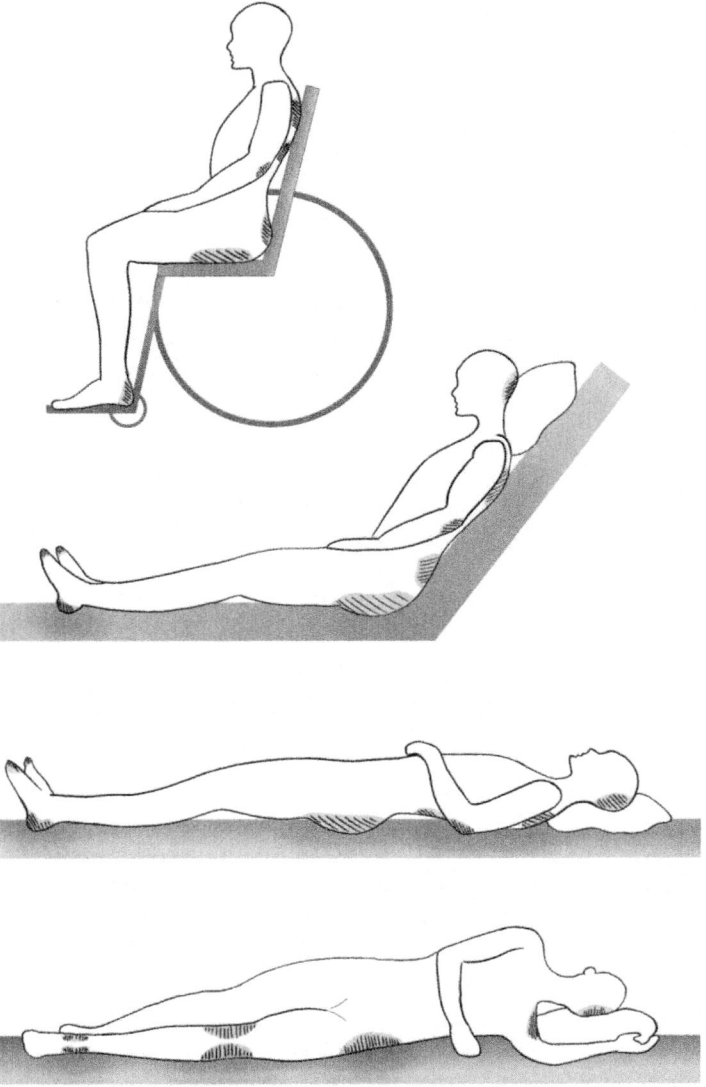

Figure 16.2 Vulnerable areas for developing bedsores.
Areas under sustained pressure, and bony areas, are at risk.

Stages of Bedsores

Bedsores are classified into four stages depending on their progress
and the level of damage:

1. In the first stage, the skin turns red, is unbroken, and may be painful when touched. With darker skin, the area may appear blue or purple, rather than red. The affected area may look like a blister. When you press on it with your finger, damaged skin does not turn white like skin with normal blood flow would under light pressure.

2. In the second stage, the top layer of the skin is broken or peeled off. The skin is red and is slightly depressed compared to the healthy skin surrounding it. The area may look like a ruptured blister, and the surface of the sore may be slightly wet from discharge.

3. In the third stage, the sore is deeper, larger, and a white layer of subcutaneous fat is visible. It looks like a small hole with dead yellow tissue at the bottom.

4. In the fourth stage, the most advanced stage, the sore has progressed deep enough to expose muscle, bone, and tendons. A significant amount of dead tissue is visible at the bottom of the wound, which can appear yellow, or dark and dry. If left untreated, the wound continues to grow wider and deeper.

Treating Stage 1 and 2 Bedsores

In the first and second stages, treatment is usually done by the caregiver at home. Treatment includes eliminating pressure from the affected area, cleaning and dressing the sore, preventing infection, managing pain, and providing proper nutrition.

- Wash the wound area at least twice per day. Use lukewarm boiled water and mild soap with low pH.

- To dry, place a paper or cloth towel on the affected area to absorb moisture and then remove the towel. Just dab with the towel. Do not wipe or rub the area because the skin may break and turn into an open, second stage sore.

- Have the patient lie down and, with the help of a reading lamp or a hair dryer, gently heat the affected area for approximately twenty minutes. This helps blood circulation at the wound site and also dries the wound of any discharge. Be careful not to burn the skin. Never leave the patient unattended under a heating source.

- Gently apply a mixture of zinc oxide ointment and milk of magnesia on the affected area. You may use sterile petroleum jelly, or other ointments as recommended by your pharmacist, instead. The key is to prevent the wound from getting dry or contaminated so it can heal on its own.

- You can cover or bandage the wound with medicated adhesive dressing specially formulated for bedsores. Consult with your pharmacist.

Treating Stage 3 and 4 Bedsores

As a bedsore grows deeper and more advanced, its treatment grows more difficult. Treating a bedsore in the third and fourth stages may require specialized medical interventions, including professional nursing care, physiotherapy, reconstructive surgery, and in some cases, orthopedic and neurosurgery.

SEIZURE AND DEMENTIA

After a couple of years, Mom's seizures began. Sometimes, while sitting, her eyes would roll up into her head, and she'd pass out. Then after a couple of minutes, she'd wake up again. One time, as she was about to sit down, she fell, as if thrown to the ground.

A seizure is a burst of abnormal electrical activity in the brain with physical symptoms such as severe muscle contractions, tremors, jerking limbs, blank stares, or eyes moving from side to side. Seizures often lead to falls. They are usually accompanied by changes in behavior, emotions, or consciousness.

Seizures can occur for any number of reasons. In adults, causes include head trauma, brain tumors, vascular or infectious diseases, drug interactions and side effects, and abnormal levels of sodium or glucose in the blood.

Epilepsy is a chronic disorder characterized by recurring seizures that are not caused by some treatable medical condition, such as alcohol withdrawal, electrolyte imbalances, or hypoglycemia. Epilepsy is more common among the elderly and young children.

Prevalence of Seizures in Dementia

Seizures are more common in patients with dementia, especially in those with Alzheimer's disease or vascular dementia, than in healthy older adults. About 12 to 26 percent of dementia patients experience at least one seizure, usually in later stages of dementia progression.

Seizures are also seen in patients with prion diseases and frontotemporal dementia. In contrast, patients with Parkinson's disease dementia do not seem to be at a higher risk of developing seizures compared to healthy individuals.

For dementia patients, impaired balance and the potential for falls adds to the risk factors for head trauma, and consequently seizures, especially in the late stage of dementia progression.

Treating Seizures

> *My mother had multiple seizures for about a year, but with the help of medication, her seizures are now under control.*

Seizure attacks, which are often short-lived, must be distinguished from other brain disorders, such as migraines and transient strokes. Laboratory techniques such as imaging procedures may be used as diagnostic tools. For dementia patients, diagnosis and treatment of seizures involve special challenges.

- The presence of cognitive impairment may prevent accurate and timely diagnosis. Caregivers and doctors may confuse seizures with other symptoms of dementia.

- Since most dementia patients are among the elderly, age-related changes in drug absorption and metabolism may alter the effectiveness of anti-seizure medications.

- Some anti-seizure medications may have side effects that make the symptoms of dementia worse.

Most seizures can be controlled with medication. The key is to strike a balance between controlling seizures and managing the drug's side effects.

What To Do In Case of a Seizure

The primary concern during a seizure is to keep the patient safe and comfortable.

1. Stay calm and ask others to stay calm.

2. Keep the patient safe. Remove objects that may cause them injury as a result of their convulsions and other involuntary movements.

3. If the patient is on the floor or in bed, turn them on their side so their mouth is toward the floor to prevent saliva or vomit from entering their windpipe and creating a suffocation hazard.

4. Loosen or remove any clothing (like shirt collar, necktie, and scarf) or jewelry that may constrict the patient's neck. Put a pillow under the patient's head.

5. Seizures are frightening experiences for patients and those around them. The patient may be confused or embarrassed by what has happened. Reassure them that they are safe, and when they are fully conscious and aware, let them know what happened in simple, short sentences.

6. Make a note of the time and duration of the seizure. It is important that the person who witnessed the seizure be able to describe the incident precisely and in detail to the doctor, as the patient may not remember the attack themselves.

7. Contact your doctor at first opportunity.

What to Avoid During a Seizure

- Never forcefully restrain the patient's arms and legs during a seizure. Restraining the patient does not stop their seizure, and may cause dislocation or fracture of arms or legs, which may necessitate surgery afterwards.

- Never force the patient's mouth open, and never put a foreign object, including your hand, in their mouth. Keep in mind that a rupture of the tongue heals relatively easily and on its own, but if you break the patient's jaw, or seriously hurt your own fingers, surgery may be the only option.

- Never give the patient any food, liquids, or medication until they are fully conscious. Otherwise, the material may end up in their windpipe and lungs, causing infection or suffocation.

When to Call Emergency Medical Services

Call your local emergency services if you encounter any of the following:

- Recurring seizures
- Seizures that last more than five minutes
- Breathing problems
- High fever and heatstroke
- Physical injury to the patient during seizure
- Patient not regaining normal levels of consciousness and awareness
- If seizure is caused by fluctuations in blood sugar in a diabetic patient.

17 | PREVENTIVE CARE

Soon after a diagnosis of dementia, one must attend to pending or postponed medical procedures. Take care of any dental work, adjustment to dentures, prescription eyeglasses, hearing aids, as well as routine preventive care.

Preventive care remains an ongoing concern throughout the course of dementia progression. Painful or damaged teeth and gums impair the patient's ability to eat and drink. Impairment in vision and hearing makes it harder for the patient to make sense of the world around them. Addiction complicates everything, making behavioral issues even more intractable.

Such issues add to the complexity of care and, if not properly managed, may develop into full-blown health crises down the road. It is therefore vital to plan for ongoing preventive care throughout the course of dementia and tend to it with diligence.

HEARING IMPAIRMENT AND DEMENTIA

There is a direct correlation between hearing loss and dementia among the elderly: those with mild hearing loss are twice as likely to develop dementia as those without hearing loss, and those with severe hearing loss are five times as likely. Hearing loss also intensifies the symptoms of dementia. It disconnects patients from the social world around them, deprives them of communication, and speeds up their descent into apathy and isolation.

It is difficult for a patient with dementia to recognize that they may be developing hearing loss. They may not be able to express it, know what to do about it, or decide that they need to see a doctor. It is up to the caregiver to watch for signs of hearing impairment and seek medical attention soon after the discovery.

Types of Hearing Impairment

The process of hearing requires the proper functioning of three main components:

- The mechanical structure of the ear responding to pressure changes in the air

- The nerves carrying the signal to the brain

- The auditory center in the brain responsible for making sense of the stimuli.

Problems with the mechanical structure of the ear may be treatable by medication or surgery, while problems with nerve transmission may be managed with a hearing aid or cochlear implant. Hearing problems due to damage to the auditory center of the brain, however, cannot be corrected through such interventions.

Problems with the auditory center of the brain may lead to auditory processing disorders where the patient becomes unable to understand the meaning of what they hear, even though they have good hearing. Dementia patients often suffer from auditory processing disorder: they appear to be hard of hearing, but will not benefit from hearing aids.

Time to See a Doctor

Usually, hearing loss develops gradually, so it's tempting to ignore it. However, since hearing loss is one of the factors contributing to the onset of dementia, and worsens cognitive decline afterwards, it is important to deal with it promptly.

- Take the patient to an otolaryngologist (ear/nose/throat specialist) at the first signs of hearing problems.

- Take with you the patient's medical records and the list of their medications.

- Inform the doctor of the patient's dementia.

Audiometry

The doctor may prescribe an audiometric test, especially if the problem seems to be caused by nerve damage. Most people with hearing loss wait too long before taking an audiometric test, typically about ten years after the onset of hearing impairment. That's ten years during which any associated cognitive decline may go unchecked.

Another reason not to delay a visit to the doctor is that audiometry is best undertaken when the patient is still able to understand and cooperate with the doctor and the technical staff. Once dementia advances beyond a certain point, the chances of performing an accurate audiometric test will be very small.

- Before taking the patient for an audiometric test, inform the office about the patient's dementia and schedule the appointment for when the center is not very busy. Crowded places and long wait times can make the patient anxious, which can affect the accuracy of the audiometric test.

Based on the results of the audiometric test, the doctor may prescribe a hearing aid.

Hearing Aids

Make sure that the patient wears their hearing aids properly.

- Ensure that the hearing aid fits well in the patient's ear. Check and adjust the hearing aid settings regularly, as the patient may tamper with them.

- Consider investing in a digital hearing aid. These types of hearing aids are small, can be almost hidden inside the ear, and their settings cannot be easily changed by the patient.

- Follow the manufacturer's instructions for cleaning and maintenance of hearing aids.

- Hearing aid batteries usually last from four to seven days. Keep spare batteries available so you can replace the batteries when necessary.

- Keep the prescription for the hearing aid in a safe place in case you have to replace it.

Using a hearing aid does not mean that the patient will regain their past verbal ability and can communicate like they used to. You'll still have to be mindful of the patient's cognitive limitations as you try to communicate with them.

VISION PROBLEMS

Although vision problems can develop for a variety of reasons, most are age related, and the most common types can be corrected with one or two pairs of prescription eyeglasses. Other types of vision problems, however, are more difficult to correct, and may involve conditions such as cataract (clouding of the eye lens), glaucoma (damaged optic nerve), macular degeneration (deterioration in macula, part of retina), and stroke or other damage to areas in the brain responsible for processing visual information.

In dementia, vision problems resulting from the deterioration of brain structures are common and a source of special challenges for patients and caregivers.

When to See a Doctor

Dementia patients may not recognize that they have vision problems. They usually cannot seek help, express their discomfort, or decide to see a doctor. So, it is up to you to keep a watchful eye for any issues and take action when necessary.

Take the patient to see an ophthalmologist as soon as you notice any vision problems. Notify the doctor of the patient's dementia and show them a list of the patient's medication.

- The best time to see a doctor is early on, while the patient is still able to understand and cooperate with the doctor. With advancing dementia, this window of opportunity closes rapidly.

- Before taking the patient for a vision evaluation, inform the office about the patient's dementia. Make the appointment for a time when the center is not very busy. Crowded places and long wait times can make the patient anxious and less cooperative.

- If the patient suffers from cataract or other complications and needs surgery, inform the surgeon of the patient's dementia so the procedure and anesthesia can be planned accordingly.

Selecting Prescription Eyeglasses

Make sure that the patient has proper eyewear. Inadequate vision, including glasses that do not fit properly, may cause a variety of behavioral issues, such as anxiety, confusion, aggression, and headaches, and generally result in a lower quality of life.

- The patient may need two sets of glasses, one for reading and working with their hands, and the other for distance vision, like watching TV.

- If the patient needs two sets of glasses, opt for two separate glasses with different shapes and colors, rather than a single pair with bifocal or progressive lenses. Over time, it will become increasingly difficult for the patient to use bifocal or progressive lenses.

- Select lightweight frames and have them fitted with unbreakable and scratch-resistant lenses.

- Equip eyeglasses with straps so the patient can carry them easily and with less chance of misplacing them. Choose straps that are not too long so they don't get tangled up with doorknobs, faucets, and other fixtures and furniture.

- Always keep the patient's eyeglasses clean.

- Keep the patient's prescription in a safe place so you can replace their eyeglasses if they are lost or damaged.

- Take the patient to see an ophthalmologist once a year, for as long as possible. Keep their eyeglasses in good condition and their prescriptions up to date.

Oral Care

Think about the steps required to brush your teeth: you must pick up the toothbrush, pick up the toothpaste tube, open the lid, gently squeeze the tube and place a small amount of toothpaste on the toothbrush, close the lid, and put the tube back in its place, while still holding the brush. Then comes the impossible task of maneuvering the brush against your teeth, all the while controlling foam and saliva from getting on your clothes or spilling on the floor. Then you have to spit, rinse, put the brush back in its place, dry yourself with a towel, and on and on. And you must do all that in the right order.

Not long into the course of dementia progression, patients lose the ability to remember and keep track of the steps involved in maintaining good oral hygiene. Over time, they find it increasingly difficult to engage in these tasks, even with the help of their caregiver. Eventually, the patient will stop caring about oral hygiene, and this responsibility, like so many others, will fall completely on the shoulders of the caregiver.

Dangers of Tooth and Gum Disease

Inadequate oral hygiene can lead to pain and discomfort in the mouth, and can bring on more serious, even life-threatening conditions. Problems with teeth and gums may aggravate dementia symptoms in many ways.

- The pain associated with tooth decay and gum disease may worsen the patient's confusion and anxiety, leading to new and more severe behavioral issues.

- Tooth and gum pain may make it harder for the patient to chew their food, resulting in indigestion. The pain may discourage the patient from eating enough, resulting in malnutrition.

- Tooth decay may lead to gingivitis.

- Decaying teeth, swollen and bloody gums, and infections of the mouth contaminate the patient's saliva and can turn an inevitable aspiration (inhalation of food stuff) into a full-blown lung infection.

Daily Oral Care

Help the patient with daily oral hygiene to ensure that they maintain chewing ability and enjoy a higher quality of life for as long as possible.

Brushing Teeth

- Help the patient brush their teeth at least twice a day, the last one being just before bedtime.

- Watch for mistakes while the patient is brushing. Due to memory problems, the patient may invent or substitute steps, or use the wrong objects or materials. For example, the patient may use shaving cream instead of toothpaste.

- Use short and clear instructions. Don't say: "Brush your teeth." Instead, remind the patient of the steps involved and wait for the patient to complete each step before announcing the next. Say: "Hold the toothbrush in your hand; place toothpaste on the toothbrush; now begin brushing."

- Use the "look at me" technique: explain each step in short, simple sentences, then do the step yourself and wait for the patient to copy your action.

- Try different toothbrushes to find one that works best. Electric toothbrushes usually don't work very well, since their noise tends to increase patients' anxiety and confusion. A patient who is already accustomed to using an electric toothbrush, however, may feel fine using one.

- Sooner or later, the patient may forget how to spit out after brushing or may not be able to rinse their mouth. Although swallowing small amounts of toothpaste is not a big deal, you may still want to switch to brushing without toothpaste in order to prevent the patient from drooling and messing up their clothes.

Cleaning Dentures

If the patient wears dentures:

- Remove dentures after each meal and clean them with a toothbrush and water.

- Every night, soak dentures in a mild denture-soaking solution.

- Clean the patient's gums, tongue, and oral cavity with a small gauze or soft toothbrush.

When the Patient Cannot Brush Any More

Eventually, the patient will depend entirely on you for oral care and hygiene.

- Wash your hands with soap and water each time before you brush the patient's teeth.

- As you proceed with the brushing routine, briefly explain each step to the patient.

- Be careful not to injure the patient's gums or oral mucosa.

- To prevent drooling or aspiration, especially in the late stage of dementia, you may switch to brushing without toothpaste.

Managing Oral and Dental Issues

One time, after we took out her dentures, she wouldn't let us put them back in. From then on we had to puree her meals.

Since patients with dementia are often unable to communicate their discomfort, warning signs may go unnoticed and small problems may quickly turn into big ones. It is therefore vital to stay vigilant and spring into action at the first sign of oral or dental problems.

- Carefully monitor the patient's facial expressions while eating. Watch how they chew their food. If they do not eat well, or if they frown in pain, probably they have gum or tooth ache, or their dentures do not fit well.

- The patient may gain or lose weight at different stages of dementia progression. As a result, their dentures may not fit properly and may lead to sore or swollen gums. Watch for signs of dentures no longer fitting properly and correct the problem right away.

- Sugar, whether in food, soda, or sweets, accelerates tooth decay. While you don't have to eliminate sweets altogether from the patient's diet, consider cutting back on sweets and limit them to meal times only.

- Some medications prescribed for dementia may cause dry mouth as a side effect. Insufficient saliva production may damage oral mucosa and accelerate tooth decay. Drinking more water during the day and at meal times can help. Your doctor may prescribe artificial saliva spray or gel to further help with dry mouth.

- Take good care of the patient's dentures. If dentures are damaged or lost, getting a new set can be difficult or impossible. With advancing dementia, the patient will grow unable to endure the process of getting fitted for a new set.

Visit Your Dentist Frequently

Before long, the patient's inability to follow instructions or cooperate may make it impossible to maintain adequate oral hygiene at home. Therefore, more frequent visits to the dentist are necessary to identify and treat problems in time.

- Visit a dentist at regular intervals, such as once every three months. Visits to the dentist should be more frequent after a dementia diagnosis than before.

- Choose a dentist with an eye toward the future needs of the patient. Ideally, you want a dentist who is knowledgeable and has experience dealing with dementia and has the necessary patience for the challenges that it entails.

- Check the location of the dental office and ways to access it. Stairs, inadequate parking, or long wait times may cause the patient to become restless, anxious, and uncooperative.

- Frequent, regular visits to the dentist will help detect problems early on. You and your dentist can then formulate a plan to deal with any problems, with due consideration of the patient's condition and their stage of dementia progression.

Soon After a Diagnosis of Dementia

The best time for tending to postponed dental work is in the early stage of dementia, while the patient still has the necessary cognition and can communicate and cooperate with their dentist. The more time that goes by, the harder it becomes for the patient to understand and comply with the dentist's requests. Before long, any dental work other than simple inspections and cleaning becomes impractical.

- Visit your dentist as soon as possible after a diagnosis of dementia. Let them know about the diagnosis, ask them to anticipate the patient's short- and long-term dental care needs, and schedule the needed work in an expeditious manner.

- If the patient needs a filling, a crown, a bridge, or a new set of dentures, get them done as soon as possible.

- If the patient suffers from gum disease, such as gingivitis, and needs surgery to correct it, do not start any major dental work until the gum disease has been resolved. Consult a periodontist before doing any major dental work.

Surgery and Anesthesia

Surgery and anesthesia present difficult questions for family members caring for a loved one with dementia. First, there is a real possibility that the operation and anesthesia will worsen the patient's cognitive decline. The decision to operate or not has to balance the risks against the potential gain. Then there are the difficult questions of whether such interventions are in the best interest of a patient who might be going through the final phases of their dementia journey.

These are very hard decisions indeed. The one guiding light in all such considerations remains, as always, the best interest of the patient.

The Risks of Anesthesia

It is common for people who undergo anesthesia to experience various side effects after the procedure, including memory and other mental and behavioral disorders.

- Around 19 to 41 percent of individuals who undergo general anesthesia exhibit cognitive symptoms similar to dementia. This condition is known as post-operative cognitive dysfunction (POCD) and may last from days to weeks, or even months, after surgery, especially in older patients.

- With dementia, post anesthesia complications can be more severe, last longer, and can worsen the patient's ongoing cognitive decline. A person at the early stage of dementia and with mild symptoms may develop severe symptoms of cognitive decline as a result of surgery and anesthesia.

Is Surgery Really Necessary?

The decision to go ahead with surgery depends on a number of factors, including the patient's physical and mental condition, and their stage of dementia progression. Before you agree to surgery, make sure that your loved one really needs the operation.

- Surgery is categorized into elective, semi-elective, and emergency. Even emergency surgery may not be the right course of action, depending on the specifics of the patient and their condition. It's often wise to get a second opinion before making a decision.

- Discuss the operation with the medical team that is involved in your loved one's care, including the patient's neurologist. Make sure that all relevant concerns are addressed and the approach with the best likely outcome is selected.

- Do your research, ask questions, and get informed about the timing and urgency of any proposed surgery, its risks versus benefits, and the likelihood of experiencing significant POCD given the patient's individual situation.

- For a patient in the early stage of dementia, the likelihood of bouncing back after the operation tends to be relatively high. The better the patient's physical and mental condition going in, the higher the chances that they will come out okay.

- In contrast, for a patient in the late stage of dementia and mostly bedridden, the risks of operation and anesthesia may outweigh any potential benefits.

This is a difficult decision, and you and your family may second-guess the decision countless times, well into the future. Nevertheless, you must make a decision and live with the consequences. Remember that not making a decision is itself a decision.

The Decision to Operate

- If the patient needs surgery and anesthesia, the best time to do it is in the early stage of dementia progression. During this period, the patient has the necessary physical and mental ability to prepare for, undergo, and successfully recover from surgery.

- Be sure to inform the surgeon and the anesthesiologist about the patient's dementia, so they can select the right type and amount of anesthetics to be used, and properly evaluate the risks of its interaction with other medications that the patient might be taking.

ADDICTION AND DEMENTIA

Prolonged substance abuse is associated with a higher risk of cognitive decline in later years. Once dementia is present, substance abuse can accelerate its progression and worsen its symptoms. Substance abuse also makes it harder to suspect or diagnose dementia, as loved ones may attribute dementia symptoms to addiction. Proper diagnosis may require clinicians with expertise in both addiction and dementia.

Reduce Risks Associated With Addiction

Memory problems, impaired impulse control, and other issues increase the risks of poisoning and overdose in dementia patients. Moreover, as people's tolerance for drugs and alcohol naturally declines with age, it may take relatively small amounts of drugs or alcohol to cause an overdose in an elderly patient.

- Inform your doctor of any alcohol, tobacco, or other substance use. Follow your doctor's instructions regarding the timing of medications to reduce the risks of interaction with alcohol or other substances that the patient may be using.

- Prevent overdose. Patients may not remember how many drinks, pills, or cigarettes they've had. Keep drugs and alcohol out of view and out of reach. Give the patient a set amount at a time and according to a set schedule.

- Do not leave cigarettes or ashtrays lying around. Dementia patients often put objects in their mouth, in the same way that toddlers do. The patient may ingest cigarettes or cigarette butts and end up with nicotine poisoning.

- Stay with the patient while they smoke to ensure safety. A lit cigarette or pipe is a fire hazard. The patient may forget and leave a lit cigarette in bed or drop it in a wastebasket, just as they might forget and leave their eyeglasses in the fridge.

- Patients may turn to drugs or alcohol to cope with anxiety and depression. Use touch, activity, kind words, and togetherness to soothe the patient's anxiety and keep them engaged with life.

Quitting and Withdrawal

Quitting is difficult and has its risks. The physiological process of withdrawal may cause or affect other medical conditions, and may even lead to life-threatening situations. Because of these risks, quitting should be done under medical supervision, where withdrawal symptoms can be properly managed.

- Look for drug and alcohol treatment facilities with detox programs designed for individuals with dementia.

Seek Medical Advice Early On

Dementia complicates addiction, and the presence of addiction makes caring for a loved one with dementia even more challenging. Specialists with expertise in both addiction and dementia can help guide you through the next steps. Depending on the specifics of the patient's situation, your doctor may recommend addiction treatment or strategies to help you manage the patient's addiction through the course of their dementia.

18 | BATHING

Regular bathing is a central part of any hygiene program, and remains so during the course of dementia progression. Bathing is essential to warding off disease and other health problems, such as skin irritations, rashes, and infections.

During the early and most of the middle stage of dementia progression, bathing is a source of stress and consternation for the patient and their caregiver. Arguments, crying, even aggressive behavior are often part and parcel of the bathing ritual, as the patient refuses to surrender to the necessity of this basic hygiene task. Even into the late stage of dementia, when the patient is wheelchair bound or bedridden, they may still resist the idea of bathing, and get anxious or aggressive at bath times.

After the bath is a different story. Being clean and properly groomed is a great morale booster for the patient and the rest of the family. Seeing the patient with trimmed nails, tidied hair, cleanly shaven (if appropriate), and wearing clean clothes offers a breath of fresh air in the otherwise drab daily routines of life with dementia.

BARRIERS TO BATHING

Patients' experience of bathing changes with dementia. What was once a refreshing and relaxing activity devolves over time into a stressful and overwhelming sensory and cognitive burden. The noise of the running shower and the exhaust fan, the beads of water pelleting their skin, the impossibility of getting the water temperature right, not knowing where to begin or what to do next, and a myriad of other problems conspire to make for a truly unpleasant bath-time experience.

Physical Barriers to Bathing

- Is the bathroom cold?
- Does the noise of the fixed showerhead annoy the patient?
- Is the running shower making the patient anxious?
- Is the floor slippery and the patient is afraid they may fall?
- Do they have difficulty adjusting the water temperature?
- Is the patient suffering from some pain or discomfort?

Psychological Barriers to Bathing

- Does the patient believe that they already took a bath or don't need one?
- Are they worried that they will not remember how to bathe?
- Are they afraid of being alone in the shower?
- Do they feel vulnerable when they take their clothes off?
- Does your presence in the bathroom embarrass the patient?
- Is the patient suffering from depression or apathy? Do they lack motivation to do anything?

BATHING ALONE

Gradually, I had taken over the household responsibilities from Mom, but she still managed to bathe on her own. I used to feel so happy when I'd see her cheeks rosy after a shower. One day I checked up on her in the shower. She was scrubbing her face so hard that I had to intervene. "Okay, now wash your body," I said. She started scrubbing her face again. "Mom, wash your body." But again she went back to scrubbing her face. That's when I realized she had been only washing her face all this time.

It may be a while before you have to be physically present during bath times. Keep in mind that even while the patient is able to manage on their own, dementia makes it increasingly difficult for them to do so safely. It is important to take precautions early on to prevent accidents before there is one.

- Adjust the water heater temperature to a setting that reduces the risk of scalds.

- If you have the option, install a faucet with separate hot and cold controls, rather than a single-lever combination faucet. Patients usually find it easier to manage separate controls.

- Install a handheld showerhead. They are more comfortable to use and less noisy.

- Install a bath seat or shower chair with backrest and armrests, so the patient can sit while bathing.

- Remove unnecessary and unsafe items like razors from the bathroom.

- Make sure that the patient cannot lock themselves in the bathroom.

- Keep a watchful eye on the bathing process to make sure that the patient does it safely, correctly, and thoroughly.

BATHING TOGETHER

Today is our bath day. I have prepared the bathroom and all the necessary items. The water heater is on. I have turned on the heater in the bathroom. Towels, clothes, and soap are all set. The only missing parts are you and me. We have to bathe to smell good. Today we are having lunch at your favorite restaurant.

Preparing for a Bath

- Choose the best time for bathing, when the patient is not tired and is more cooperative. If they are anxious or resist strongly, postpone bathing to another time.

- Prepare the bathroom in advance so it is warm and inviting.

- Make sure the water heater temperature is at a setting that reduces the risk of scalds.

- Prepare all the needed items beforehand so you won't have to leave the patient alone during the bath. Your attention must be fully dedicated to the patient during bathing times.

- Remove unnecessary and unsafe items like razors from the bathroom.

- Play the patient's favorite music or sing a tune that they are familiar with and enjoy.

- Set a reward for bathing, such as going for a drive, ice cream in the park, or dinner at their favorite restaurant.

During a Bath

- If the patient is uncomfortable with you in the bathroom, do not undress them completely right away. Alternatively, you can partially cover their body with a towel.

- If the patient does not allow you to undress them before going into the bathroom or the shower, do not force the issue. As their clothes get wet, the patient will be much more amenable to removing them one by one.

- Have the patient hold a small towel or a bath sponge in each hand to keep them occupied. Otherwise, they may grab your hand and disrupt the bathing process.

- In a friendly tone and with short sentences, announce every step just before doing it. After each sentence, pause briefly so the patient can process the information.

- If the patient can do some steps on their own, let them do it. Use the "look at me" technique to help the patient remember what to do: explain each step in short, clear sentences, then do the step yourself and wait for the patient to copy your action.

- Use a handheld showerhead instead of a fixed one. With a handheld showerhead, you can manage the washing more easily and the patient will not have to suffer through the noise and indiscriminate splashing of a fixed showerhead.

Drying Afterwards

- Use bathing time as an opportunity to check the patient's entire body for skin injuries, rashes, red spots, and other signs of a pressure sore developing.

- Do not rub a towel on the patient's skin. Just put the towel on their skin, or dab the skin with it. Over time, their skin will grow fragile and may break with the slightest stretch.

- Before dressing the patient, sit them in a chair. Put some zinc oxide cream or baby powder on the areas where skin folds over skin, like under the abdomen, to prevent skin irritation.

- Comb the patient's hair and put a little makeup or aftershave, as appropriate, on their face. This will improve the patient's mood, as well as that of the rest of the family.

Bathroom Wheelchair

Later in the course of dementia progression, you will have to bathe and dry the patient while they sit in a bathroom wheelchair. You may need the help of a second person for dressing the patient.

- You can undress and prepare the patient in a convenient staging area while they are seated in the bathroom wheelchair, then roll the wheelchair into the bathroom.

- To undress the patient, first lower their pants, then ease the patient into the bathroom wheelchair. Finish undressing the patient while they are comfortably seated in the wheelchair.

- Engage all four brakes on the bathroom wheelchair during prepping and bathing. Otherwise, it will move when you are busy handling the patient, creating a fall hazard.

- When leaning the patient forward to wash their back, stand in front of the wheelchair to prevent it from tipping over or the patient falling forward.

- Make sure the patient's tailbone is not in contact with the chair, especially the hard edge of the hole in the seat. The hole in the seat makes it easy for the tailbone to rub against the hard edge of the seat, setting the stage for a pressure sore.

Getting Help During Bath Times

- Do not lock the bathroom door from the inside. Others should be able to get to you promptly if there is any mishap and you need help.

- Establish a procedure for other family members to check up on you, should the bathing process take longer than usual.

- Set up codes for communicating from the bathroom. For example, using a wireless buzzer, one ring can indicate that washing is finished and others can use hot water for dishes or laundry, while two rings can indicate that you need help and someone should come to the bathroom right away.

BATHING IN BED

Bathing in bed may seem daunting at first, but with a little planning and the right equipment, it can be a relatively easy and smooth process.

- Before attempting a bed bath, you'll need to have mastered the procedure for changing bed sheets while the patient is lying in bed and unable to cooperate with you (described later in this chapter).

- The following procedures are described in reference to a hospital bed. A hospital bed can make bathing in bed a lot easier by allowing you to adjust the height of the bed to a comfortable level so as to minimize strain on your back.

Preparing the Supplies

Prepare what you will need ahead of time so you won't have to leave the patient alone during bathing. You'll need:

- Two buckets (one for soapy water, one for rinsing)
- One waterproof sheet or a large towel to keep the bed dry
- A few washcloths or sponges
- A few bath towels
- Soap, shampoo, and moisturizing lotion
- Makeup items or shaving supplies
- A set of clean clothes.

Safety First

- Keep the room warm. Close the windows and turn up the heat as necessary. Keep the patient covered at all times. Uncover each area only when it is being washed.

- Safeguard the patient's privacy. Close the door and draw the curtains. Cover the patient with a towel before undressing them. Only undress the areas that are to be washed.

- Have someone present to help you, especially if you have to roll the patient onto their side. Raise the bed's guardrails to ensure the patient cannot fall out of bed.

- Raise the bed to a comfortable height so you don't strain your back.

- Spread a waterproof sheet or a large towel under the patient so the bed does not get wet. Follow the procedure for changing bed sheets later in this chapter.

- Use warm water for washing. Maintain a water temperature range of 100 to 110°F (38 to 43°C). The water should feel comfortably warm to your elbow.

Wash, Rinse, Dry, Inspect

- Fill two buckets with warm water, one for soaping up a sponge or washcloth, and the other without soap for rinsing. Be prepared to change the water at least once during the course of bathing.

- Wash with a wet washcloth and soapy water. Rinse using another washcloth and clear water. Dry the area before moving on to the next area.

- To dry, spread a towel on the area, pat it, and remove the towel. Do not rub the towel on the patient's skin, as it may cause the skin to break.

- Wash a single area at a time. Uncover the area, wash, rinse, and dry, then cover it up again before moving on to the next area.

- While washing, inspect the patient's entire body for signs of skin rash, scratches, and red spots which can be a prelude to pressure ulcers.

Wash in Order

- Start with the cleanest areas of the body, and progressively move on to areas that are less clean.

- Wet a washcloth without soap. Gently wipe one eyelid from the inside and moving out, and then pat it dry. Repeat on the other eyelid, using a different part of the washcloth.

- With soap and water, wash the face, ears, and neck. Rinse and dry before moving on.

- Wash one side of the body, and then the other side. Wash the shoulder, arm, and hand, on both sides, then the chest and belly, including the belly button, then the hip, leg, and foot on one side, then the other. Wash one area at a time with soap and water, then rinse, dry, and cover before moving on to the next.

- Pay special attention to areas with skin-on-skin contact or folds, such as the armpits, abdomen, belly button, and between the toes. These areas must be clean and dry to prevent skin irritation and fungi growth.

- To wash the patient's back, first roll the patient onto one side and wash one side of their back, and then roll them onto the other side and wash the other side of their back.

- Wash the genital area at the very end. Change the bath water, and use a clean washcloth. First wash the genitals, and then the buttocks. Wash from front to back.

- If the patient is able to help, let them wash the genital area themselves. Bend their knees for better access. Make sure they wash from front to back.

Washing the Head

For a wash with water and shampoo, you'll need a source of running water, such as a bottle or a kettle, and a large waterproof sheet and a bucket to collect the rinse water.

- Adjust the bed so it is completely horizontal.

- Pull the patient to the upper edge of the bed so their head is at the top end of the bed. Take care not to stretch or break their skin in the process.

- Roll the waterproof sheet at one end and place it under the patient's neck. Put the other end of the sheet into the bucket on the floor, underneath the patient's head. Raise the sides of the sheet at the upper end to create a channel to guide rinse water into the bucket below.

- Wash the patient's head with water and shampoo, massaging their scalp in the process. Then rinse, taking care not to splash water onto the patient's eyes and face. Finally, dry their hair with a towel.

Washing With Dry Shampoo

Alternatively, you can wash the patient's hair with a special dry shampoo. This type of shampoo does not require water or rinsing, and is typically used when a patient is hospitalized or cannot get a regular bath for a short period of time.

Grooming

Put moisturizing lotion on fragile areas of the patient's skin, like their shins and toes. Remove the wet towels and the waterproof sheet, and then help the patient to get dressed. Comb their hair and apply a gentle makeup or aftershave as appropriate.

CHANGING BED SHEETS

Eventually, you'll have to change bed sheets, underpads, and diapers while the patient is lying in bed and unable to cooperate with you. The procedure in all these cases is the same, and involves turning the patient onto one side, and then the other.

- Changing bed sheets is a two-person job: one person to roll the patient to their side, and another person to spread and remove the bed sheet.

- Always roll the patient toward you. Stand guard to prevent the patient from rolling farther forward and off of the bed.

Removing Bed Sheets From Under the Patient

1. Turn the patient onto their side.

2. Roll the free side of the bed sheet toward the patient as far as possible.

3. Turn the patient over the rolled sheet to the other side.

4. Remove the sheet.

Adding Bed Sheets While the Patient Is in Bed

1. Prepare the bed sheet by rolling up about a third of the sheet lengthwise.

2. Turn the patient onto their side.

3. Lay out the sheet on the bed, with the rolled side of the sheet along the patient's body.

4. Turn the patient over to their other side, onto the sheet.

5. Spread the rolled part of the sheet.

Replacing Bed Sheets

To replace bed sheets, you'll have to perform the removal and placement of bed sheets at the same time.

1. Prepare the replacement sheet by rolling up about a third of the sheet lengthwise.

2. Turn the patient onto their side.

3. Roll the free side of the old sheet toward the patient, then lay out the new sheet in its place, with the rolled side as close to the patient as possible.

4. Turn the patient over to their other side, onto the new sheet.

5. Remove the old sheet completely, and spread the rolled part of the new sheet in its place.

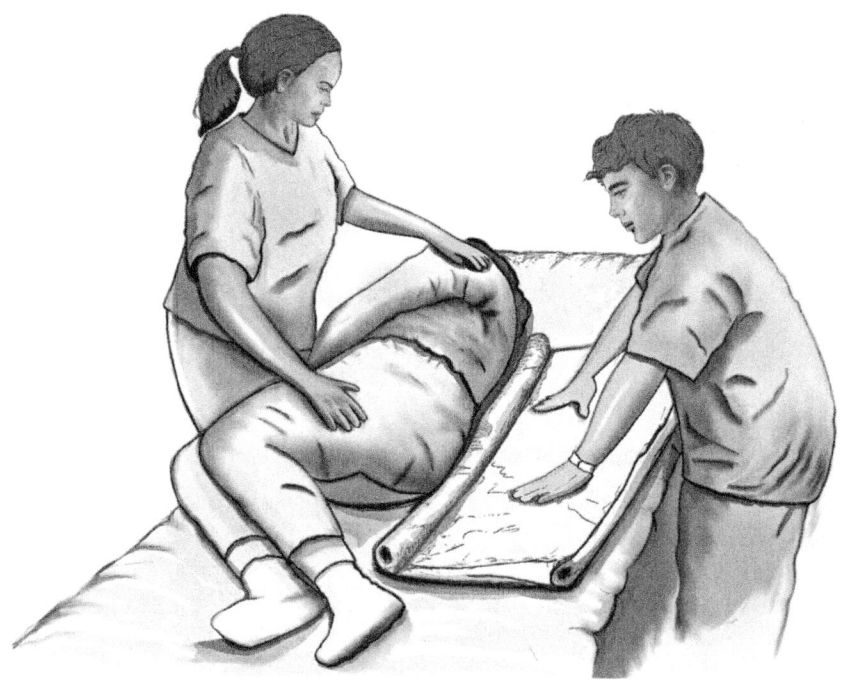

Figure 18.1 Changing underpads and bed sheets.
Roll the patient toward you and stand guard for safety.

19 | MOBILITY AND BALANCE

Few patients maintain balance and mobility into the late stage of dementia progression. Most lose the ability to keep their balance toward the end of the middle stage and need more help and support from their caregivers for walking, sitting down, and getting up.

As the patient grows less active over time, it falls on the caregiver to help keep the patient's muscles, tendons, and joints healthy and mobile. Eventually, simple stretching and massage will be the only means of exercising the patient's limbs, which must be tired and stiff from countless hours of sitting immobile or lying in bed.

PRESERVING JOINT MOBILITY

The patient's range of motion gradually diminishes over time, mainly due to inactivity, arthritis, and related issues. To preserve joint mobility and range of motion for as long as possible, schedule regular stretching exercises as part of the patient's daily routine, and take special precautions during prolonged sitting and sleeping to prevent limbs from growing stiff and locking up.

Stretching Safety

Include stretching exercises at least once per day, such as upon waking up, to help increase blood flow to muscles and preserve mobility in the joints. Gentle stretching also helps wake up the nervous system and get it primed for balance and mobility. Practice waking up the nervous system every time after prolonged sitting or sleeping.

All the usual warnings regarding stretching safety apply here as well. When you help the patient through their stretching routine, take care to not overstretch or injure them, especially if the patient is unable to communicate their pain or discomfort to you.

- Adjust the stretches over time to match the patient's ability.

- Take care not to put excessive pressure on the patient's joints.

- Look for signs of discomfort in the patient's face or demeanor. Do not continue to stretch through pain or discomfort.

- Do not rush through the stretching routine, and do not crank the patient's arms and legs through each repetition.

Range of Motion Routine

When the patient is no longer able to sit or stand, you'll have to perform the stretching routine for them. The following is an example routine for a bedridden patient. Do around ten repetitions for each stretch. You can devise similar routines if the patient is able to follow while sitting in a chair or standing up.

1. With the patient lying in bed, raise their arms vertically toward the ceiling. Then open them wide to the sides.

2. Lay the patient's arms down along their body on both sides. Then, without folding the arms, bring them all the way up above their head.

3. Raise the patient's arms vertically toward the ceiling. Then stretch each arm over the patient's chest toward the opposite side. Hold this position for a few seconds.

4. Bend the patient's right leg from the knee. Bring the knee up toward the abdomen. Hold for a few seconds, then bring the leg back to its resting position. Repeat for the left leg.

5. Bend both legs from the knees and bring them together up toward the patient's abdomen. Hold this position for a few seconds, then bring the legs back to their resting position.

6. Bend both legs at the knees, with the soles of the feet resting on the mattress. Gently push the knees apart into a butterfly position, hold for a few seconds, then bring them back together.

Joint Care During Sleep

-   During sleep, put a small pillow on either side of the patient under each armpit, between the arms and the body. This is to prevent the arms from getting stiff or locking in place on the sides of the body overnight.

-   When the patient is sleeping or lying on their side, put a small pillow between their knees. This helps reduce lateral stress on their hips, which can cause them to stiffen. It also helps prevent bedsores from developing at the knees.

-   Use a boomerang pillow to better support the patient's head and shoulders when the patient is lying on their back. When sleeping on their side, rest only the patient's head on the pillow.

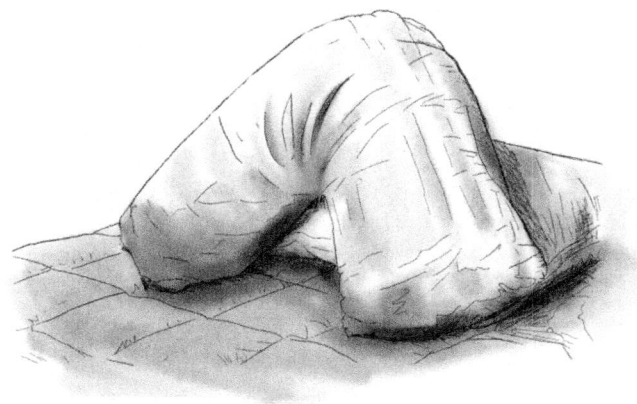

Figure 19.1 Boomerang pillow

Physical Activity

With the onset of dementia, patients tend to grow inactive and sedentary rather quickly. It is important to keep the patient active and moving in order to preserve their quality of life for as long as possible and slow down the rate of their cognitive decline.

Dementia does not spell the end of physical activity in the patient's life. Many activities can be modified to suit the patient's evolving abilities. Physical activity remains essential to the general well-being of the patient throughout the course of dementia progression. It is also an effective means of reducing behavioral problems, including anxiety and confusion.

Exercise and Dementia

Simple, natural exercises do not require special equipment. They're also effective at improving the patient's mood, as well as that of their caregiver.

- Include a variety of physical activities in the patient's regular daily schedule.

- Include simple exercises in natural settings, such as walking in a park and light gardening.

- Include regular morning stretches in the patient's daily routine.

Intensity and Duration

- Schedule more strenuous activities for the early hours of the day when the patient is fresh and has more energy.

- Adjust physical activities to match the patient's ability and stamina. The patient's ability will naturally vary from day to day, and generally tapers off over time with advancing dementia.

- Avoid excessive and monotonous exertion. Remember that the goal is to improve the quality of life of the patient. How fast, how far, and how long are irrelevant questions.

Rest and Recovery

- Keep it fun and relaxing. When walking in the park, allocate time to relax on a bench and enjoy the environment; watch streams flowing, birds singing, and children playing. Refuel with a healthy snack, like an apple or a banana.

- Plan for rest after exercise. Schedule a ten-minute rest on the park bench or a nap upon returning home. But, do not schedule long naps in the afternoon because they may interfere with a good night's sleep.

- Ensure proper hydration during and after exercise. Consider the intensity and duration of the exercise routine and the ambient temperature. Drink plain water and limit the consumption of carbonated and sweetened beverages.

Sprinkle Physical Activity Throughout the Day

My mother is in the middle stage of dementia and is quite sedentary. We have to work very hard to get her to walk a few steps with the help of a walker or a cane. When we finally get her to walk, she curses and grumbles the whole time.

Over time, walks will gradually get shorter and rest periods longer. Eventually, impaired balance makes it too dangerous to take the patient for a walk outside. To keep the patient active, help them walk short distances at home.

- Sprinkle exercise throughout the day. Take the patient to the bathroom every hour. This helps with incontinence and injects some regular exercise in the patient's daily routine.

- If the patient resists the idea of exercise, do not try to reason with them. Just hold their hand gently and use gestures that indicate you're asking them to get up. Then walk them aimlessly around the room, and into and out of other rooms. Use the same technique to take the patient to the bathroom every hour.

LOSS OF BALANCE

She'd stop at the shadow of a streetlight on the ground, thinking it was a ditch. On an incline, I'd hold her hand, and we'd walk up together with small steps, like little children. When going down a few steps, I'd have to go in front, hold both her hands, and help her down, one step at a time. It'd take us around fifteen minutes to walk down four or five steps.

Patient safety takes on different dimensions over the course of dementia progression. During the early stage, the patient needs little reminders for safety, such as "Watch your step," "Use the handrail," or "Mind the bump on the road." Over time, you may have to hold their hand to prevent falls or have the patient wear a gait belt for you to hold on to. Toward the late stage of dementia progression, the only safe and practical means of transport is a wheelchair.

Sudden Loss of Balance

My grandmother needs to hold my hand when we go for a walk. She squeezes so hard that it gets painful pretty quickly.

The challenge of walking with dementia increasingly comes down to the looming risk of a sudden loss of balance and a subsequent fall. When walking with the patient, stay vigilant and in physical contact with them so you can feel a sudden loss of balance and can help stabilize them in time.

- The patient may fall without any prior warning signs. They may be walking just fine, and then suddenly and without any obvious reason, may lose their balance and fall.

- While walking with the patient, gently caution them about immediate situations requiring their attention, like approaching stairs or using a handrail.

- Hold hands while walking. Early in the course of dementia, walking hand in hand is usually enough to keep the patient out of trouble and help them with minor balance issues. With advancing dementia, however, you'll need to maintain a more robust contact with the patient for safety.

- For a more robust hold, start by taking the patient's dominant hand (usually the right hand) in yours in a handshake position and then immediately turn it into an arm wrestling handhold. Turn your body to face in the same direction as the patient, and use your free hand to hold the patient around the waist.

- Alternatively, you can use your free hand to hold the patient's arm or elbow, instead of their waist. This technique works early on, when the patient still has relatively good balance.

- Use a gait belt to help stabilize the patient while walking. With your free hand, hold on to one of the loops on the belt to ensure that you can keep the patient steady in case there is a sudden loss of balance.

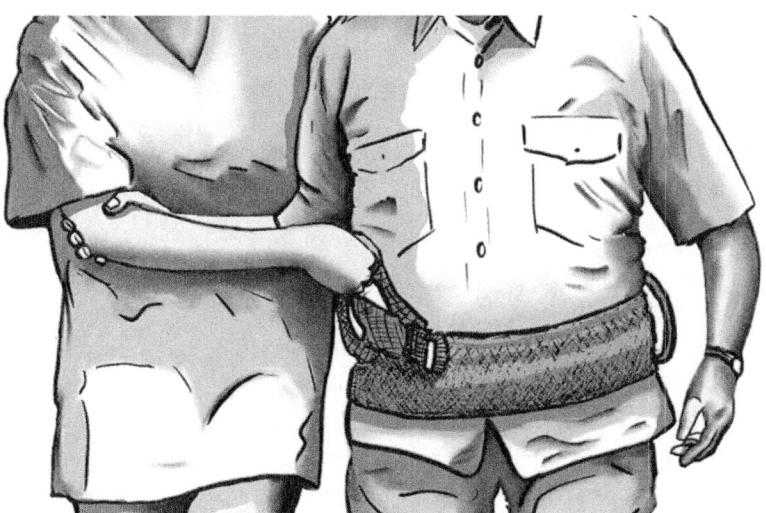

Figure 19.2 Using a gait belt for support.
Hold on to one or two of the loops for safety.

In Case of a Fall

A gait belt can help you salvage a potentially disastrous situation. If the patient suddenly loses their balance and you cannot keep them from falling, a gait belt can make the difference between a controlled descent to the ground versus an unrestricted fall.

1. Use your grip on the gait belt to gently lower the patient to the ground.

2. Once on the ground, gently arrange the patient's limbs so they are in a natural position and not twisted or under pressure.

3. When you are ready, help the patient to stand up again, getting assistance from someone else, if needed.

4. If you cannot lift the patient and immediate assistance is not available, make the patient as comfortable as possible. Stay calm while you figure out what to do next.

Loss of Balance When Sitting

My mom suffers from Parkinson's disease and dementia. A few days ago she was sitting on the bed, when she suddenly lost her balance and fell onto the floor.

A sudden loss of balance and a subsequent fall can happen at any time: when the patient is standing or walking, or when they're sitting in a chair, on the edge of the bed, or on the toilet.

A sudden loss of balance is especially dangerous in small, confined spaces, such as a small bathroom. If the patient falls, it will be very difficult to maneuver in the confined space to help them get up, especially if you need additional help or if the patient gets wedged between the toilet and the bathroom wall.

- Equip the toilet and the patient's chair with armrests and backrest to provide extra support and reduce the chances of the patient falling.

Using a Walker for Support

As the patient's ability to learn and remember diminish over time, it becomes progressively harder to learn new skills, such as using a walker. To assess whether the patient can learn to use a wheeled walker, try it at home first where you can control distractions and noise. If the patient can use the walker comfortably at home, then you can try it in a quiet area outside your home. As always, stay vigilant to prevent any potential loss of balance and falls.

TIME FOR A WHEELCHAIR

One nice afternoon, we were getting ready for some coffee and cake in the backyard. Everyone was managing their own task, and one person was handling the wheelchair. When she turned for a moment to close the door behind her, the wheelchair started rolling, slowly. A few feet behind, someone screamed, but it was too late. The wheelchair reached a step and slowly went over. My wife, strapped in the chair, unable to speak or even raise her hands to break the fall, hit the hard mosaic face-first. In the commotion that followed, she didn't say anything, couldn't say anything. She didn't even moan or cry. She just watched helplessly as we ran around in panic, trying to salvage the situation.

By the late stage of dementia progression few patients are able to walk anymore. Most lose the ability to maintain their balance toward the end of the middle stage and need special care for movements and transfers. Starting in the middle stage, and through the late stage, the primary tool for patient transportation will be a wheelchair.

Choosing a Wheelchair

Choosing a wheelchair is an important decision, since it will affect so much of life in so many subtle ways, both for the patient who will spend countless hours sitting in it, and for the caregiver who will push, lift, and operate it for months to come.

- Buy a suitable wheelchair as you notice the need approaching. Do not postpone this task until the last minute because you may have difficulty finding a wheelchair with the exact specs that you need.

- A standard wheelchair has large rear wheels for easy handling on bumpy terrain. You just need to raise the front wheels slightly and push the wheelchair over bumpy areas on its rear wheels. Bathroom wheelchairs typically have four small wheels and can only be used over smooth surfaces.

- Choose a wheelchair that is made of lightweight material, such as aluminum, and whose wheels and footrests are easily detachable for easier handling. Make sure you can easily lift the wheelchair and that it fits in the trunk of your car.

- Make sure the wheelchair fits through important doorways in your home, including the doorways to the bathroom and the patient's bedroom.

- If the patient cannot propel the wheelchair on their own, you can remove the hand-rims to make the wheelchair narrower by about two inches. This may be enough for the wheelchair to fit through narrower doorways.

- Equip the wheelchair with a good cushion to prevent pressure sores from developing on the patient's buttocks and tailbone.

Wheelchair Safety

Exercise care and vigilance when operating the wheelchair, especially since the patient will not be able to assist you in its safe operation or warn you of looming dangers.

- Always apply the brakes on both wheels before attempting to transfer the patient to or from the wheelchair. Otherwise, the wheelchair can move and create a fall hazard.

- Always apply the brakes on both wheels when you are standing in one place. All it takes is a moment of distraction for the wheelchair to start rolling on its own on the subtlest of inclines.

- When climbing a ramp, stay behind the wheelchair and push it up the ramp. When going down a ramp, walk the wheelchair backward down the ramp. Do not walk down a ramp with the wheelchair in front, as the wheelchair may escape from your grasp or the patient may fall forward.

- Equip the wheelchair with a seatbelt, and use it consistently to prevent the patient from rolling forward and falling off.

Clearing Obstacles

Operating a wheelchair involves more than just pushing it. You'll have to negotiate small steps, edges of rugs and carpets, or small pebbles capable of stopping the front wheels of the wheelchair dead in their tracks.

Climbing Up a Small Step

1. Position the wheelchair near the step, facing it.

2. With the help of the foot levers at the back of the wheelchair, tilt the wheelchair to raise the front wheels off the ground.

3. Push the wheelchair forward until the front wheels are on top of the step. Lower the front wheels so they rest on the step.

4. Push the wheelchair forward until the back wheels are touching the step.

5. Raise the back of the wheelchair and place the back wheels on the step.

To make sure the front wheels can safely be lowered on the step, you can combine steps 3 and 4, that is, push the wheelchair forward until the back wheels touch the step before lowering the front wheels.

Climbing Down a Small Step

To move the wheelchair down a small step, follow the above procedure, but going backward, and in reverse order:

1. Position the wheelchair near the step, with its back toward the step.

2. Step down on your own first before attempting to bring the wheelchair down.

3. With the wheelchair's front wheels resting on the step, lower the back wheels gently down the step onto the ground below.

4. Pull the wheelchair away from the step, maintaining the tilt of the wheelchair until the front wheels are fully off of the step.

5. Gently lower the front wheels to the ground.

Stepping Over an Obstacle

To clear a small barrier, you'll have to "step over it" with the wheelchair, first moving the front wheels over the obstacle, and then the back wheels:

1. Tilt the wheelchair to raise the front wheels off of the ground. Then push the wheelchair forward, and lower the front wheels on the other side of the obstacle.

2. Push the wheelchair forward until the back wheels are against the obstacle.

3. Lift the back wheels just enough to clear the obstacle. Then push the wheelchair forward, and lower the back wheels on the other side of the obstacle.

Pushing the wheelchair forward on its front wheels is a delicate maneuver since even a small pebble on the path is enough to stop the front wheels suddenly. Any time the wheelchair is leaning forward, if possible, keep one hand on the patient's chest or shoulder to help stabilize them in their seat. This is easier to do when the back wheels are resting on an obstacle less than two inches high, so you can just push the wheelchair forward and off of the obstacle with one hand.

- Avoid leaning the wheelchair forward or pushing it forward on its front wheels.

- Keep one hand on the patient's chest or shoulder to stabilize them in their seat.

- Use a wheelchair safety belt to keep the patient securely strapped in the wheelchair.

20 | PATIENT TRANSFERS

Patient transfers, such as from bed to wheelchair, are difficult maneuvers that must be carried out several times per day in later stages of dementia progression. Correct technique is essential in order to prevent injury to the caregiver or the patient.

To attempt these maneuvers, you must be physically healthy, with no medical complications in your neck, shoulders, lower back, pelvis, and knees. Any pre-existing medical or health issues, coupled with an incorrect lifting technique, may cause irreparable damage to you, and create a fall hazard for both you and the patient.

Problems with sitting down, getting up, and balance tend to appear over time, giving you the opportunity to practice your technique while the patient still has the ability to assist in carrying their own weight. By the time they are unable to assist you anymore, you should have mastered the necessary techniques.

SITTING DOWN AND GETTING UP

At some point, usually in the middle stage of dementia progression, the patient will have difficulty sitting down and getting up, and will need special help. Typically, problems with sitting down tend to appear earlier than problems with getting up. The right furniture and the proper techniques can make the process easier and safer for both patient and caregiver.

Choosing the Right Furniture

The right furniture can greatly improve the ease and safety of patient transfers. A chair that is low to the ground and allows the patient to sink in is much more difficult to work with than a chair that sits up relatively high and has good cushions. A chair that can slide during patient transfers is extremely dangerous and a fall hazard.

- Choose a chair or sofa that is heavy or backed up against a wall so it cannot move during transfers.

- Select a chair or sofa that sits higher than regular furniture and has hard foam cushions. Lifting a patient sunk in a soft chair, or placing them in a low chair, is very difficult and will put extra strain on your back.

- When transferring the patient to or from a wheelchair, place the wheelchair close to and at a 45-degree angle to the bed, sofa, or chair. If possible, position the wheelchair in such a way that it cannot move backward. Apply the brakes and remove footrests from the wheelchair.

- To ease patient transfer in and out of bed, use a hospital bed and adjust its height as necessary for safe transfers.

Guiding the Patient Onto a Chair

My mother resists sitting down. I think she's afraid of falling. I sit down to show her how, and sometimes she follows. Sometimes I have to repeat sitting down several times before she follows suit.

By late middle stage of dementia progression, the patient will have difficulty lowering into a chair or onto the toilet. The backward movement inherent in the sitting maneuver makes it harder for the patient to trust that they will not fall.

1. Take the patient's dominant hand (usually the right hand) in yours and with your other hand behind their back, gently walk the patient to the chair.

2. When you are close to the chair, gently pivot the patient 180 degrees so their back is toward the chair.

3. While still holding the patient's dominant hand, and with your other hand supporting their back, gently move the patient backward until the back of their knees touch the front edge of the chair.

4. Turn to face the patient, and hug them. Hold your hands together around their lower back. Hold this position for a few moments to comfort and relax the patient.

5. Keep your knees in front of the patient's knees to ensure stability and to prevent their knees from coming forward during the next step.

6. Bend your knees to lower your center of gravity, keeping your knees in contact with the patient's. With the back of their knees still against the chair, the patient will bend their knees and start to sit down.

7. Lower the patient gently into the chair and continue to hold them in a hug for a few moments to help them relax.

When lowering the patient onto a chair, if they understand you and can follow verbal instructions, ask them to put their hand on the chair's armrest and help you lower them into the chair.

LIFTING SAFETY

There are three main components in every transfer:

1. Lifting the patient

2. Pivoting and otherwise adjusting the patient to line up with the target location

3. Lowering the patient onto the target location.

All three components must be carried out with proper technique in order to prevent injury. Improper raising and lowering of the patient may put undue strain on the caregiver's lower back and shoulders, risking injury. Improperly executed pivoting may result in twisting the patient's knees or ankles, causing fractures. By far the greatest risk, however, is that of losing balance in the process and falling together.

How to Lift a Load Safely

Lift with your legs and knees, and not with your back. Do not bend your back, and avoid any twisting motion during the lifting process or while carrying a load.

1. Stand close to the object you want to lift, with feet apart about the width of your shoulders. You'll want to hold the object as close to your center as possible when lifting and carrying it.

2. While keeping your back straight and your face and chest facing directly forward, bend your knees to lower your body to a comfortable position to grab the object.

3. Hold the object close to your center and, with the help of your knees and legs, rise slowly. Engage your core and keep your back straight to prevent undue strain on your lower back.

4. After standing upright, if you need to face a different direction, gently and with small steps turn your entire body in the desired direction. Do not turn by twisting your body left or right while carrying a load.

5. When you are ready to put down the object, follow the above steps in reverse order. Continue to keep your back straight so as to avoid putting pressure on it.

LIFTING THE PATIENT

Over time, the patient will have increasing difficulty understanding and complying with your requests. They will have a harder time cooperating when you ask them to hold your hand or put their foot forward. Eventually, they will be unable to stand up or assist in carrying their own weight in any way.

Transferring a patient who is unable to cooperate or assist in the process requires all your attention and focus. The slightest distraction or momentary carelessness can have severe consequences for both you and the patient.

- If you have difficulty lifting the patient, consider using a hoist as described later in this chapter. Using a hoist takes more time but reduces the risks of injury to both patient and caregiver.

- During manual transfers, the patient may grab your hands or cling to you out of fear of falling. To keep the patient from disrupting the transfer process, have them hold a towel or a soft ball in each hand.

How to Lift the Patient Safely

The technique for lifting a patient is an extension of the technique for lifting any other load. Use your knees and legs to lift the patient, while keeping your back straight.

1. Stand close to, and facing, the patient. Stand with your feet apart about the width of your shoulders. For better balance, you can put one foot farther back than the other.

2. Bend your knees and lower your center of gravity, keeping your back straight.

3. While directly in front of the patient, slide the patient closer to the edge of the bed or chair, but not so close that they risk sliding off of the edge. Lean the patient a little forward onto you, and make sure that their feet are firmly on the floor.

4. Brace your knees against the patient's to keep their knees from wobbling left or right, or buckling.

5. Clasp your hands together just above the patient's lower back. Lift the patient by straightening your knees, while simultaneously pulling the patient close to your center.

6. Once you are standing upright with the patient securely in your arms, hold for a moment or two to allow the patient to adapt to the new posture.

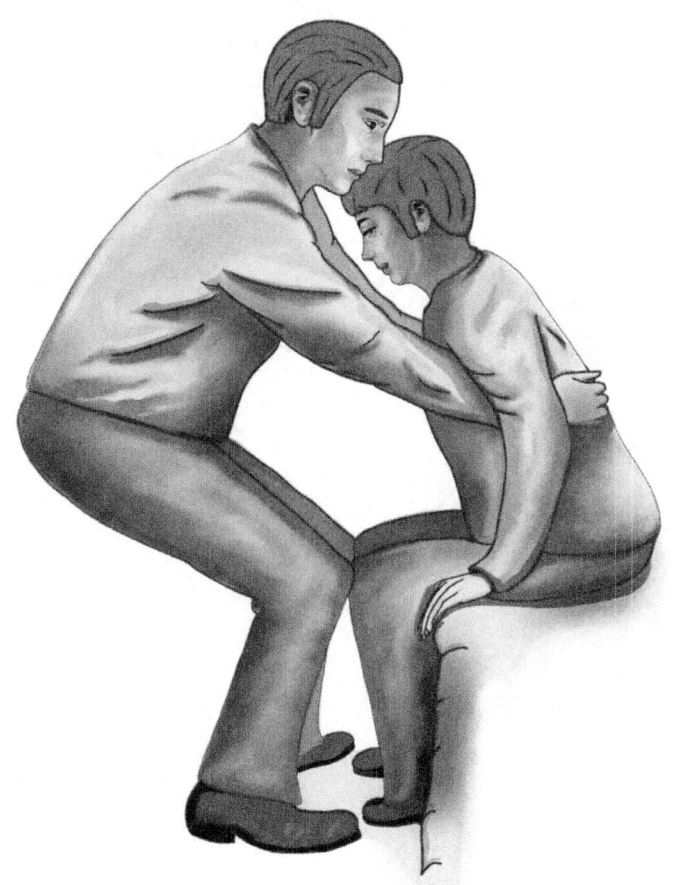

Figure 20.1 Helping the patient to stand up.
Clasp your hands behind the patient's back; lift with your legs.

Using a Transfer Belt

You may find it more practical to lift the patient with the help of a gait or transfer belt. A transfer belt provides a better grip during the lifting process, and may reduce strain on the patient's skin as you lift them. A transfer belt is especially helpful if you have difficulty reaching around the patient to clasp your hands behind their back.

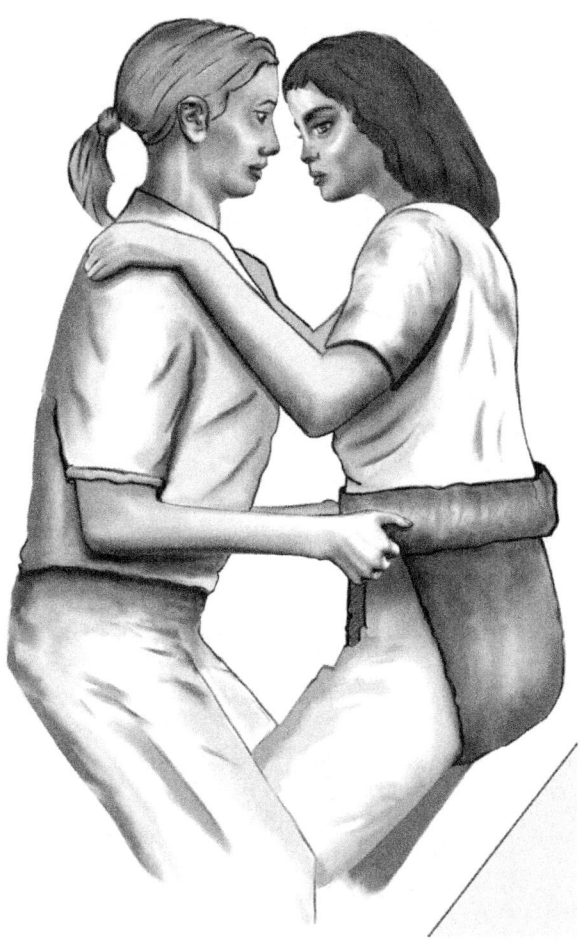

Figure 20.2 Lifting with a gait or transfer belt.
Brace your knees against the patient's knee for support.

Getting the Patient to Straighten Up

In later stages of dementia progression, the patient may not readily straighten their knees or straighten at the hips as you lift them. With a little help, however, the patient will often be able to stand up and carry much of their own weight.

- As you lift the patient, support one or both their knees from the side with yours to keep their knees from wobbling left or right, or buckling.

- Alternatively, if the patient does not readily straighten their knees upon standing up, position one or both your knees in front of theirs so that when you lift the patient, their knees straighten against yours.

- Once in standing position, pull the patient's hips toward you to help the patient straighten up against your body. You may do this by gently pulling in the patient's hips with your hands just above their tailbone.

Pivoting to the Target

Having lifted the patient, you must now turn them in the proper direction and move them back a little until they are in a position where they can be safely lowered onto a chair or other target. Follow the procedure below if the patient is unable to walk.

- Once you are standing upright with the patient securely in your arms, turn with the patient in the desired direction by shifting from one foot to another in small, controlled steps. Do not try to pivot the patient in one or two large steps as that can put excessive stress on their knees, ankles, and back, causing injury.

- To help the patient turn with you, shift their weight to one leg and, with the help of your foot, gently slide the patient's free foot in the desired direction. Then shift the patient's weight to their other leg and repeat the process.

- Using your foot, turn the patient's free foot a little after each slide so that the patient's feet remain in a natural position relative to the body at all times.

- Put socks or suitable slippers on the patient's feet to make it easier for them to slide and pivot in place, reducing strain on their knees and ankles.

SITTING UP AND LYING DOWN

At some point in the middle stage of dementia progression, the patient will need help getting in and out of bed. The first step in helping the patient out of bed is to help them sit up in bed.

Sitting Up in a Hospital Bed

A hospital bed can greatly aid the process of sitting up from a lying position, thanks to its adjustable back and height. You can simply raise the back to a near-sitting position, then swivel the patient on their buttocks.

1. Raise the back of the bed to a 45-degree angle. Adjust the height of the bed to slightly below your waist level. Remove any supporting pillows from under the patient's knees.

2. Place one arm behind the patient's shoulders, and your other arm under their bent knees. Bend your knees to lower your center of gravity, and keep your back straight. On the count of three, sit the patient upright while simultaneously pivoting the patient on their buttocks in a single controlled swivel so they end up sitting on the edge of the bed with their feet on the floor, facing you.

3. While the patient is sitting on the edge of the bed, adjust the height of the bed again, this time so that the patient's feet rest fully on the floor. Maintain a secure hold on the patient to prevent them from rolling or sliding off the bed.

Sitting Up in a Flat Bed

To help the patient out of a flat bed, first roll the patient to their side, and then help them sit up on the edge of the bed.

1. Place one hand behind the patient's shoulder and the other hand behind their hip or thigh on the side farthest from you. Roll the patient onto their side, toward you. Take care to not pull on the patient's limbs or skin.

2. With the patient lying on their side facing you, place your arm behind the patient's knees, and gently move their feet off the edge of the bed.

3. Place one arm behind the patient's shoulders, and your other arm on the patient's back or hips for additional support. Bend your knees, keep your back straight, and hold the patient firmly. On the count of three, use your legs to raise the patient to a sitting position in a single smooth motion.

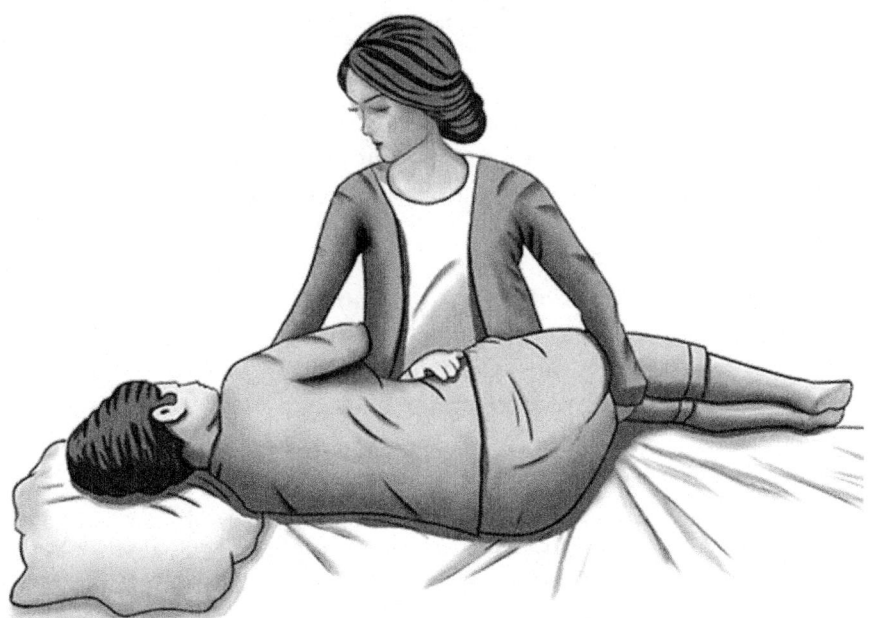

Figure 20.3 (a) Helping the patient to sit up on the bed.
Roll the patient to their side and slide their feet off of the bed.

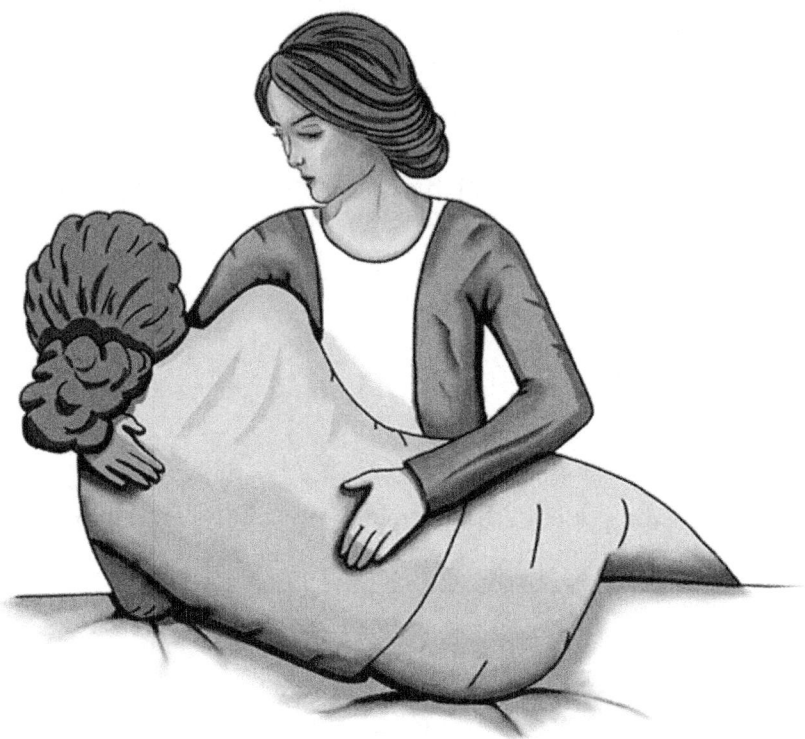

Figure 20.3 (b) Raising the patient to a sitting position.
Hold the patient firmly and raise them in one smooth motion.

Lying Down

The procedure for helping the patient to lie down is the same for both a regular bed and a hospital bed, and is the reverse of the procedure for sitting up in a flat bed. Still, a hospital bed can aid the process by virtue of its height being adjustable.

1. If the bed is adjustable, make sure the back of the bed is horizontal. Adjust the height of the bed as necessary so the patient can sit securely on the edge of the bed.

2. Maneuver the patient to a standing position by the bed so the backs of their knees are touching the bed. Lower the patient onto the bed, like you would onto a chair.

3. If the bed is adjustable, raise its height to your hip level to reduce stress on your back in the next step. Maintain a secure hold on the patient so they don't roll over, slide, or fall.

4. Place one arm behind the patient's shoulder and your other arm under the patient's knees. Bend your knees and keep your back straight. On the count of three, lower the patient to their side, while simultaneously helping their knees up to reduce stress on the patient's hips and back. Slide the patient's feet onto the bed.

5. Roll the patient onto their back and straighten their limbs as appropriate. Adjust the position of the patient on the bed as necessary.

BED TO WHEELCHAIR

During patient transfers, as in any other care procedure, describe each step to the patient, even if they can no longer understand what you say. Speak in short, simple sentences and announce each step before doing it. Prompt the patient with simple requests, like "Stand up," "Put your foot there," and so on.

The step-by-step announcement can help orient you and the patient through the process, and may enable the patient to participate and help in small ways. It also helps instill in the patient a feeling of being cared for with empathy, rather than a feeling of being handled like an object.

Transferring to Wheelchair

1. Clear the surroundings of small rugs, extra furniture, toys, or any clutter that can create a fall hazard.

2. Place the wheelchair next to the bed at a 45-degree angle. Apply the wheelchair brakes and remove the footrests.

3.   Remove any blankets and supporting pillows from around the patient. Adjust the bed and the patient's position as necessary for safe lifting.

4.   Following the proper procedure for patient transfer, lift the patient from the bed, pivot as necessary, and lower into the wheelchair.

5.   Fasten the wheelchair safety belt to prevent the patient from sliding or falling off.

6.   Install wheelchair footrests back in their position, and place the patient's feet on them. You can now release the wheelchair brakes and move it safely.

WHEELCHAIR TO CAR

If possible, install in your car a passenger swivel seat that can slide partway out of the vehicle for easier transfer. Your car's manufacturer may be able to make the necessary modifications, or you can hire someone to do it for you. You'll probably need to use a smaller car seat in place of the original one to make room for the swivel mechanism.

Additionally, you can use a swivel cushion to make it easier to swivel the patient on the car seat. These cushions are made of two separate layers connected in the middle by a wheel that turns on an axis, enabling the two layers to turn independently of each other.

Transferring to Car

1.   Open the car door, and place the wheelchair at a 45-degree angle to it. Apply the wheelchair brakes and remove the footrests.

2.   Swivel the car seat, and slide it out of the car. If your car is not equipped with a swivel seat, transferring the patient in and out of the car is still possible, but a little more difficult.

3. Following the proper procedure for patient transfer, lift the patient from the wheelchair, pivot as necessary, and lower onto the car seat.

4. Until the car seat is back in position with the patient securely strapped in with their seatbelt on, keep your hand on the patient's shoulder for support and to keep them from falling.

5. Slide the swivel seat back to a partially extended position so you can help the patient's legs into the car.

6. While supporting the patient with your left hand, put your right hand under their left knee and gently move their leg into the car. Then, move their other leg inside.

7. Shift the swivel seat the rest of the way into the car. Adjust the patient so they are facing forward and their feet and legs are in a natural position relative to the body.

8. Put the patient's seatbelt on.

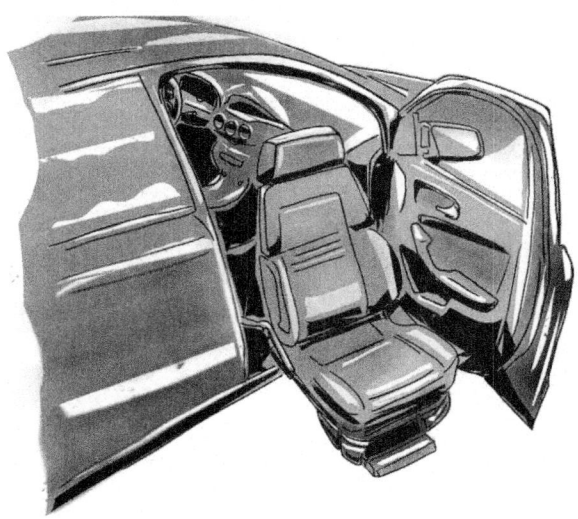

Figure 20.4 Swivel car seat

SPECIAL TRANSFER EQUIPMENT

Eventually, the patient may be unable to stand up at all; they may be unable to straighten their knees, keep their feet on the floor, or help carry their own weight in any way. At that point, lifting with a hoist may be the only viable option.

A hoist is helpful in other situations too, for example, if the patient is heavy and you cannot lift them on your own. Using a hoist takes more time than lifting the patient manually, but it is safer and may result in fewer strains and injuries to the caregiver.

- To transfer the patient with a hoist, use a sling that is specifically made for this purpose. Place the sling underneath the patient, using a procedure similar to changing bed sheets.

- Once the sling is placed underneath the patient, put the lift hooks into the holes of the sling. Lift the patient by activating the hoist's electric or manual hydraulic pump, as appropriate.

- Lifting and moving the patient with a hoist usually requires two people: one to operate the hoist, and the other to keep the patient steady and prevent unwanted swinging and rotation.

- Steer the hoist to the wheelchair or sofa, and slowly lower the patient into it. Unhook the sling from the hoist, and leave the sling underneath the patient. To lift the patient from a wheelchair or sofa and returning them back to bed, rehook the sling and follow the same procedure.

- When taking the patient to the toilet, you can use a special sling with a hole in the middle.

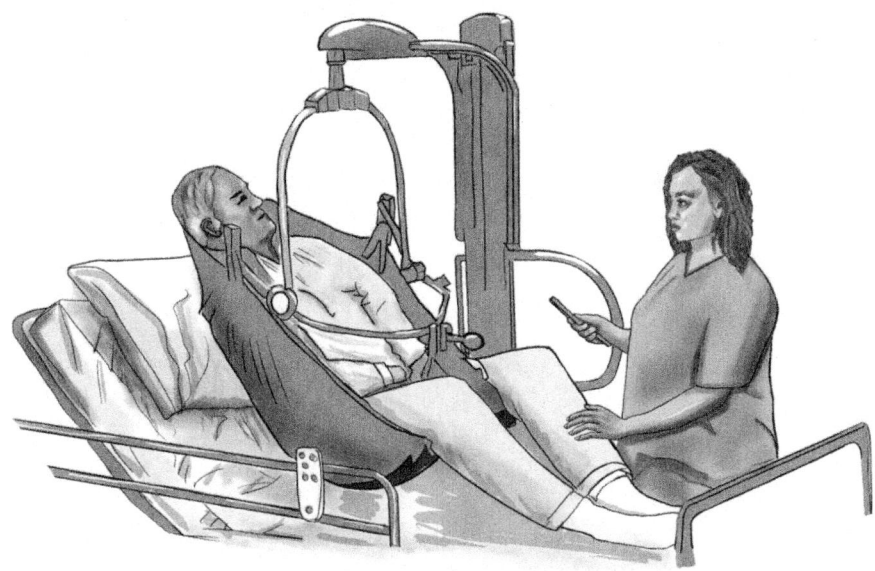

Figure 20.5 Lifting with a hoist.
Using a hoist takes more time, but is safer than manual transfer.

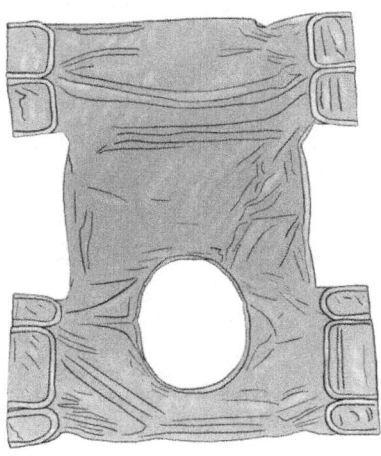

Figure 20.6 Sling for use with a hoist.
For bathroom use, choose a sling with a hole in the middle.

21 | CARING FOR THE CAREGIVER

Caring for a loved one with dementia is a commitment that spans many long years. It is not a sprint to the finish line. You simply cannot put everything on the line today, as if tomorrow will never come.

It's easy to get immersed in caring for a loved one to the point of losing sight of your own health. You should remember, however, that if you succumb to depression or burnout, the care process will, in all likelihood, collapse also. Doing right by your loved one means taking care of yourself now so you'll be around to take care of them into the future.

STAYING HEALTHY

Most caregivers experience anxiety, guilt, and depression. Don't think that you can provide perfect care, that you have to do everything on your own, or that no one can do a decent job of caring for your loved one other than you.

While you care for a loved one with dementia, you may have to take care of other commitments as well, such as a career and a family of your own. Shopping, cooking, cleaning, and other mundane demands of life will be there to fill up every available moment of every day. As you rush to look after everyone else in the family, remember that it is often the main pillar in a structure that needs the most careful maintenance.

- Don't take your health for granted. Even if you do not have any known health issues, visit your family doctor at least once a year and take care of all of your periodic health screenings.

- Listen to your body. Take any health warnings seriously. Watch for excessive fatigue, sleep problems, behavioral changes such as anger and impatience, changes in appetite, or unexplained weight gain or loss.

- Take care of your mental and emotional well-being. Relax, practice deep breathing, and meditate regularly. Consult with a psychologist, psychiatrist, or social worker when necessary.

Get Enough Sleep

Dementia often means disrupted sleep patterns for the patient and their caregiver. Inadequate sleep impairs the caregiver's ability to handle the stresses of the day, and makes the caregiver more susceptible to depression and burnout.

- Try to recharge with a short nap during the day. When scheduling a nap in the patient's daily routine, schedule one for yourself too.

- Even if you cannot fall asleep during the day, sit or lie down for a few minutes and close your eyes. Take a few deep breaths and let your mind relax. Focus on your breathing and try to relax the frown on your forehead. Five to ten minutes of meditation may be what gets you through the next hump in the day.

Have a Healthy Diet

Plan a balanced diet for both you and the patient. Try the Mediterranean diet rich in legumes, vegetables, fruits, fish, olive oil, walnuts, and almonds. Reduce consumption of fast foods.

Make Time for Exercise

It may be hard to appreciate the importance of exercise when you're exhausted all the time. However, exercise is a great way to take a break from the demands of caregiving and flush out the toxic effects of stress. Exercise also helps reset your mood and give you a renewed sense of purpose and motivation.

- Have friends and family take over caring for the patient for a couple of hours so you can take a break and go for a walk or do some other exercise or relaxing activity.

- During the early stage of dementia, while you still can, exercise with the patient. Take them for a walk in the park, go on bicycle rides, or go shopping together. Arrange activities for the patient in ways that enable you to participate along with them.

- Fit a little bit of exercise here and a little there. When an opportunity presents itself, do some stretching and light exercise to relax and calm down. When the patient takes a nap or is watching TV, use the opportunity to do some stretching or yoga.

- When putting together daily and weekly plans for the patient, do not forget to factor in exercise, rest, and recovery for yourself as well. Your planned schedule should correlate with the patient's, so you know, for example, that when the patient is taking a nap, it is time for you to do some meditation.

Stay Socially Connected

Meaningful social connections are essential for healthy living. They're even more important if you're under a lot of stress.

- Watch for creeping isolation. When caring for a loved one with dementia, you'll find that friends and acquaintances tend to drift away and lose contact over time. Make an effort to stay in touch with those who have the willingness to adapt to your new situation.

- Use all means at your disposal to connect. Use email, online forums, phone calls, and text messaging. Make a point of speaking to at least one person who does not have dementia every day.

- Join a support group. Connect with people who are on the same journey and are experiencing similar challenges. Seeing that you are not alone often helps to ease the pain and burden that you are feeling.

Manage Stress

Explore techniques to reduce or manage stress. Chronic stress may cause a variety of health problems, such as high blood pressure, headaches, and digestive system disorders. Light exercise, yoga, meditation, and breathing exercises can help manage and reduce stress.

Pace Yourself

Remember that caring for a loved one does not mean controlling everything in their life. Nor does it mean that you should do everything for them. Part of your job as a caregiver is to help the patient do things on their own, and prolong their independence wherever you can, for as long as possible.

- It's natural to feel sometimes that you won't be able to care for your loved one in the best possible way. Remind yourself that you are doing your best to provide the best care possible. Accept that your feelings of guilt are baseless.

- Include respite in your schedule. Take some time off regularly to recharge so you can continue to provide the care that your loved one depends on. Taking a break does not mean you are selfish or lazy.

- Get help from friends, family, and neighbors in day-to-day chores. You may be concerned that no one wants to help, but you will never know unless you ask. Remind yourself that it is part of your job as a caregiver to find others who can help you on this journey, and that asking for help does not mean you are ineffective or inefficient as a caregiver.

Maintain Realistic Expectations

The more you know about dementia and its progression, the less anxious you'll feel about the future. The better you understand the challenges ahead, the more confident you'll be facing them.

- Expect and accept change. With advancing dementia, your loved one will need more specialized care. Learn about the various alternatives to get the necessary help.

- Remember that the patient's behavioral changes are part and parcel of dementia and that it's the illness, not the patient, that is the driving force behind behavior issues. Don't take their behavior personally.

- It is natural to mourn the loss of physical and mental abilities of a loved one as you watch them transform into someone you don't quite recognize. Don't let the loss of the past get in the way of special moments today. Your shared story still has chapters to be written. Try to focus on the positives and make the most of the memories still to come.

I have to feed my father, take care of his personal hygiene, hold his hand when taking a walk, give him his medication, change his clothes, put him to bed... I missed my job interview because I couldn't leave home for a whole week. I'm under a lot of pressure. I remember the anger and desperation I felt at the beginning of my father's illness, and the commitment I made to my mother to care for him. It was after that commitment that I realized how deeply I loved my father, how many untold stories we had between us, and how we had been like strangers throughout most of our lives. We didn't talk much before his illness, but now we are much closer and enjoy a level of intimacy I never thought I could expect.

STRESS AND DEPRESSION

Dementia takes a toll on the emotional well-being of the caregiver. Feelings of guilt, anger, grief, helplessness, and loneliness are common among caregivers, and behavioral and psychological consequences such as withdrawal and depression are further complications. If not addressed properly, the emotional burden will have debilitating and lasting impact on the health of the caregiver, and the quality of care that they are able to provide.

Chronic Stress

A defining feature of dementia caregiving is its nonstop nature. This means that stress never stops, and the hits keep on coming, 24/7.

With each stressful event, the body undergoes physiological changes as it gears up to meet the demands of the situation. After each episode, the body needs time to clear the physiological byproducts of the stress response. This recovery period, and the return to baseline, can take up to several hours.

For a dementia caregiver, however, the recovery period is all but nonexistent. The caregiver often faces a runaway situation, where the body never receives respite long enough to clear the byproducts of stress response and recover fully.

A consequence of this chronic stress is that dementia caregivers are themselves at risk. In one study, caregivers who experienced care-related strain had a 63 percent higher mortality risk than non-caregiving controls. This makes chronic stress a primary concern for dementia caregivers.

> *My husband is restless and combative. His dementia has progressed, and his blood pressure and diabetes are worse, too. People warn me that at this pace, I will die before he does. I wonder, too, how much longer can I hold on? Is it exhaustion from the nonstop work that finally takes me, or is it the daily emotional roller coaster? For now, I just go on because I don't have any other choice.*

Signs of Chronic Stress

- Irritability
- Anxiety
- Withdrawal
- Depression
- Burnout
- Sleep issues
- Trouble concentrating
- Lack of attention to one's health

Watch Out for Creeping Depression

There's a short path from chronic stress to depression. The threat of depression should not be taken lightly. Depression is one of the most common conditions afflicting dementia caregivers and may appear at any stage of dementia progression.

What makes depression especially dangerous is the stealth with which it creeps up and engulfs its victims. Often the caregiver is not even aware of depression taking hold, until the process is well under way. By the time they realize what is happening, it's already too late.

- Task at least one friend or family member who is in regular contact with you to watch you for signs of depression. Have them sound the alarm at the first sign of a problem developing, and when they do, heed their warning.

Signs of Depression

- Persistent sadness and anxiety
- Feelings of hopelessness and despair
- Irritability
- Feelings of guilt and worthlessness

- Loss of interest and enjoyment in everyday living

- Exhaustion and lack of energy

- Problems with concentration and sound thinking

- Sleep disturbance

- Changes in appetite and weight

- Persistent issues like headaches and digestive problems

- Thoughts of death and suicide

Helping the Caregiver Cope

My brother asks how I'm doing, then walks away without waiting for a response. It's like a greeting, rather than a concern about how things really are.

If you are not the primary caregiver, you can help the main caregiver cope by helping them get things off of their chest. Have regular conversations with the caregiver. Ask follow up questions. Use effective listening techniques to draw them out and help them pour their heart out. Do not block the flow by providing solutions, or theorizing as to the reasons why something is the way it is. Just listen. Remember that your goal here is to offer up emotional support, not logical problem-solving.

- Be sincere in your desire to find out how they feel. Ask questions that cannot be answered with a simple yes or no. If you ask how they are and they answer with "I'm okay," ask more questions.

- Find ways to appreciate their dedicated effort. Ask questions like: How did Dad sleep last night? How is he tolerating his new meds? What did you do to manage his aggression? What movie did you watch last night? Was it good?

- Listen to their complaints, and pay attention to signs of stress and depression. Take warning signs seriously. Take remedial action to stop depression before it takes hold.

Let Off Steam

There will be times when you feel like you are about to explode. You feel like you are at your wits' end and unable to hold things together any more. You want to scream and break everything within your reach. This is normal, and it happens to other caregivers, too. To survive and go on, you'll have to find ways to open your safety valve and let off some steam.

- Find some solitude. Go for a drive, a walk, or a hike. Look for a change of scenery and a modicum of privacy. Find some solitude to clear your head and settle your mind.

- Let it out. Sing along your favorite tunes. Sing or speak at the top of your voice. Complain, argue, lecture the world. Pour your heart out.

- Take stock. Once you've said your piece, focus on your strengths and the positives in your life. Remind yourself that your track record for getting through bad days so far is one hundred percent.

- Let it go. Write it down, so your mind can let it go. Keep a journal. Write to get some clarity and sort through your emotions. You'll be surprised at how liberating it is to bare your soul, even if to no one in particular.

There's a worn-out mountain overlooking the cemetery where my parents are buried. I hike there a couple of times a week, when the sun is coming out and the air is still crisp. Every once in a while, I go all the way to the lonely top overlooking the cemetery below, and speak to the dead. Sometimes I call out to my mom and my dad, sometimes I scream, but most of the time I just talk, to no one in particular. Occasionally an old mountaineer passes by, one of those old guys who used to climb tall mountains all over the world. They glance in my direction, sometimes nodding hello, and go on their way. Somehow, the old guys know that the mountain is listening.

CAREGIVER BURNOUT

My mother's patience is wearing thin as she cares for my father. She regularly curses at him and has even told him to "Either get well, or die!" She still refuses to hire outside help, worrying that she can't trust anyone to do a decent job.

Caregiver burnout is a result of physical and emotional exhaustion and is a real risk among dementia caregivers. When a caregiver commits more than they are able to, or when they do not have adequate help and support, burnout is often the result. Burnout transforms the attachment and affection a caregiver feels toward a loved one to neglect and indifference, and may even lead to more severe forms of patient abuse.

- Watch for signs of burnout in the main caregiver. The symptoms resemble those of acute stress and depression.

When Is Burnout Most Likely?

My mom is very attached to me and won't leave my side. She won't stay with my siblings, even for an hour. I can't go shopping or out for a walk by myself. She has mood swings and hallucinations. She blames me for everything, all the time, and even gets aggressive at times. Sometimes I feel I just can't cope anymore.

Caregiver burnout is most likely during the period when the patient is experiencing a lot of behavioral changes. This is the period when the patient usually becomes attached to their caregiver and shadows them wherever they go. This in turn results in the caregiver experiencing all of the ups and downs of behavioral issues as they happen in real time.

- Task another member of the family with a hobby or activity that the patient enjoys. Do not engage in that activity with the patient yourself so that they start to miss it. Then, when the person who is tasked with the activity says, for example, "Let's go get some ice cream," the patient is more likely to accept.

Risk Factors for Caregiver Burnout

It's important to face dementia with sincerity and humility. See dementia, your loved one's needs, and your abilities and motivations as they are, and not as you'd want them to be. Adapt yourself to the reality of the situation because it will not adapt to you.

Unrealistic Expectations

It's tempting to hope that your loved one will recover from dementia, as they might from another illness. But, dementia is progressive, and there is no recovery. Focus instead on improving your loved one's quality of life. Find ways to manage the symptoms of dementia; discover ways to connect with the person in your care; and figure out how to better help them cope.

False Assumptions

Initially, you may feel that you can provide care for your loved one single-handedly. You might even feel that you have no choice in the matter. It is important to realize, however, that both of these are mere assumptions, and neither is true. Accept that caring for a loved one with dementia is not something you can do alone, and that you can find help, if you look for it.

Lack of Control

Lack of experience or knowledge, financial hardship, and lack of support from family and friends can all contribute to a general feeling that one no longer has any control over one's destiny. Regain a sense of control by organizing your care program around routines and schedules so you can foresee and manage issues rather than constantly having to play catch up.

Depression

It is difficult to notice the warning signs of depression when you're consumed with the demands of caregiving. As depression takes hold, it becomes even more difficult to recognize what is happening or muster the energy to do something about it. It is imperative that you stop depression early in its tracks, before it does the same to you.

Confusion in the Role of Caregiver

The caregiver who is a child or a spouse or life partner has to take on the role of a parent or guardian now. The love and affection that they're accustomed to seem to have disappeared, replaced by unreasonable demands and bizarre behavior. Remember that, although it may be difficult to decipher, your loved one still has an inner life, and the two of you still have memories to build and share together.

My husband is not the same man I knew. He shadows me everywhere I go, and yet, there is no intimacy between us anymore. He keeps making demands, and I keep trying to carry on, to keep life going for our children. Fear has taken over from the security I used to know: fear of tomorrow, of what lies ahead, fear that I won't be able to go on, or hold my family together, and fear that neither of us will be around to see our children to their future.

SAYING GOODBYE

> *We had a patient who was being discharged that morning. As the staff worked to get her ready, her son spoke to her, trying to reassure her. He spoke so softly, with such tenderness, that I made a remark about how well he took care of his mother. "I had a good teacher," he said, like he was still speaking to his mom. We see a lot of things at the hospital, but something about that picture had me scrambling for the door while I could still hold myself together.*

The story of dementia is a story of goodbyes. It's a long series of daily losses as abilities recede and more and more of a cherished soul fades behind a distant horizon. Goodbyes don't get any easier, no matter how long the journey or how many sunsets one has witnessed along the way.

A source of mounting anguish as dementia marches deeper into the advanced stage is the looming prospect of having to say goodbye for the last time. This is especially distressing for a caregiver who has been intimately invested in the care of a loved one for so long. More daunting, perhaps, is the prospect of having to shepherd a loved one through the complexities of the dying process.

Death is a part of life, and dying is a natural part of living. A little familiarity with the dying process can help demystify this fundamental part of the human experience, and to enable one to continue to provide care for a loved one with dementia, and look after the rest of the family, during this difficult period.

What to Expect

As the end of life draws near, the body begins its natural process of winding down. This process may take days or weeks, during which the patient spends more time asleep, their food and fluid intake tapers off, and their temperature and breathing may fluctuate more than usual.

- The patient spends more time asleep, and may be drowsy when awake. Do not speak loudly to wake them up. Continue to treat them gently and speak in a soft, natural tone.

- The patient's appetite and thirst dwindle. This is natural and the experience is not painful or distressing for the patient. Offer the patient food and fluids, but allow them to refuse it. Moisten their mouth and lips with a few drops of water from a mouth swab to help with dry mouth.

- The patient's body temperature may fluctuate, and their extremities may turn gray or blue, as blood circulation slows down and the body loses the ability to regulate itself. Adjust bedding and blankets as necessary to keep the patient comfortable.

- Breathing patterns may change and grow irregular. This, too, is due to blood circulation slowing down. It is not painful to the patient and usually does not require treatment. However, if the patient seems short of breath, treatment options are available, including medication, administering oxygen, or providing fresh air (by opening a window).

Hospice Care

End-of-life care requires specialized skills to care for a patient whose care needs may have grown quite complex, and for their loved ones who are going through one of the most difficult periods of their lives. Hospice care is designed to address both concerns: to provide palliative care for the patient in the final few months of life, and to provide support and care for family members during this process.

Hospice care may be provided at home or at dedicated facilities. It includes professional care, counseling and emotional support, help in finding resources and services, and help with spiritual needs. It is typically provided by a team that includes doctors, nurses, social workers, counselors, chaplains, and others.

Hospice care can provide relief to the family during the final weeks and months of their dementia journey. It ensures that their loved one is receiving proper care, while enabling the family to spend more quality time with their loved one during these precious final months.

When It's Time to Say Goodbye

The final hours and minutes are moments to spend together in love and gratitude. This is the time to ease the patient on their way, while helping others in the family onto the rest of their journey. The currency of this moment is not so much in doing or saying things, but in togetherness and being present in the moment.

- Keep the patient's environment calm and quiet. Close family and friends may be present in the patient's room, but sitting quietly while one person caresses the patient's hands.

- Speak to the patient quietly, and in a comforting tone. There is evidence that the sounds of loved ones can help bring comfort to patients in their final moments.

- Visitors may spend time with the patient alone, one at a time. They may caress the patient's hands, whisper words of love and gratitude, thank the patient for all their love and sacrifice, and ask for forgiveness.

- If you're the spouse, a child, or a close family member, tell the patient not to worry about you. Let them know you'll be alright.

> *I sat by his side and held his hand one last time. I told him what he had meant to me, thanked him for his love and kindness through the years, and asked for his forgiveness. I kissed him on the cheek and whispered in his ear: "It's okay, Dad. I know you have to go. You've done all that anyone could ask for, and more. Go when you're ready. Go, and be at peace." And just like that, he was gone.*

SUPPORT GROUPS

There's nowhere to turn to, no one who understands, and no shoulder to cry on. After my mom's diagnosis, there was a barrage of comments from friends and relatives who didn't know what to make of the situation. People felt awkward and didn't know how to behave around my mom anymore. Slowly, they abandoned us, and visits to our home became a rarity. In the final years, no one helped: no family, no acquaintance, no friend or neighbor. When I took my mom to the park, people stared, sometimes asking about her tremors and wondering out loud why we even came out of the house.

A support group can be a lifeline, a source of advice, help and encouragement, and an outlet for feelings that only those with similar experiences can truly understand. In the right group, you'll find members who share their knowledge and experience with generosity, and support each other with compassion. With the help of the right support group you can:

- Feel less lonely and learn that you are not alone

- Learn how to better manage common problems

- Reduce feelings of stress, anxiety, depression, and helplessness

- Get more familiar with what you can expect down the road

- Learn about local services and facilities.

Venues of Support

Support groups may be held one-on-one, in a group setting, or in an online forum. Some groups meet face-to-face, while others use the phone or the Internet to connect. Groups are usually managed by one or more current or former members. They may invite experts to their meetings now and again, depending on the topic being discussed.

Find the Right Group

Before joining a support group, do your due diligence. Learn about the group, their charter, their objectives, membership rules, privacy policy, and how the group is managed. Talk to your doctor about the support group that you intend to join. Your doctor likely knows about reputable groups in your area.

- Is membership free or do you have to pay a fee to join?
- Are the group's goals well defined and consistent with your needs and values?
- Does the group's manager or moderator have the necessary experience in this area?
- Are conversations among members kept private and confidential?
- Is the group's schedule compatible with yours?

Warning Signs

Common warning signs that a group is not suitable for you include:

- The group requires you to buy a product or service
- It assures you that a product or service will fully treat your loved one
- It encourages you to disregard the advice of your doctor
- It judges your work and your care plan.

Ease Your Way In

After you join a support group, take some time to get familiar with the dynamics of the group before posting questions or answers, or otherwise sharing your problems or situation. With more confidence in the sincerity of the members, you can decide when and how much to share with other members.

Exercise Good Judgment

Take the advice you receive with a grain of salt. Remember that such advice is not a substitute for medical consultation with a qualified doctor or specialist. Experiences shared in a support group may not be applicable to all cases and all patients, and may even be counterproductive or dangerous in your specific situation. In particular, any change to medications, even over-the-counter ones, should only be made with the approval of your doctor.

Stay Vigilant

Bear in mind that people you meet in a support group may not be who they claim to be. They may give you incorrect information, or may be there to take advantage of vulnerable members, financially or otherwise. Safeguard your personal information and do not divulge your phone number or address to people you don't know. Do not be quick to trust members who try to sell you something, or offer you a new treatment.

When It's Time to Leave

A suitable group is one which deals with its members' shared needs, stays true to its purpose, and does not drift into other, or unrelated, areas over time. If you find that the group's nature or direction has changed, you do not have to stay in the group.

> *I lost my mother this year. I used to think that once her journey came to an end, I wouldn't need the help of my support group anymore. When she passed, I didn't even write about it on the forum. But the more time passes, the more I find myself attached to my support group. They're my family now. I follow their journey and reminisce about my own. And I try to help others navigate the twists and turns of the road, and avoid the pitfalls that I experienced along the way.*

The Journey Goes On

There's no end to the road,
Nor is there a beginning.

The journey goes on –

The sun will rise tomorrow,
And the grass is still green.

Resources

National Associations

- Alzheimer's Association
  News, articles, local chapters, support groups
  24/7 helpline: 800-272-3900
  www.alz.org

- The Association for Frontotemporal Degeneration
  News, articles, local chapters, support groups
  24-hour helpline: 866-507-7222
  www.theaftd.org

- Frontotemporal Lobar Degeneration Association
  News, articles, local chapters, caregiver support
  www.ftlda.org

- Lewy Body Dementia Association
  News, articles, support groups
  Lewy Line: 800-539-9767
  www.lbda.org

- American Stroke Association
  News, articles, resources, support
  www.stroke.org

Government Resources

- National Institute of Health
  General health information, news, research
  www.nih.gov

- National Institute on Aging
  General health information, news, research
  www.nia.nih.gov

- National Library of Medicine
  Resources, research papers, information
  www.nlm.nih.gov

- National Library of Medicine, MedlinePlus
  Information about drugs and supplements
  www.medlineplus.gov

- Centers for Disease Control and Prevention
  Resources, information
  www.cdc.gov

Research Hospitals and Foundations

- Mayo Clinic
  News, health information
  www.mayoclinic.org

- Memory and Aging Center
  University of California, San Francisco
  Information, research news, dementia
  memory.ucsf.edu

- Stanford Health Care
  Information on dementia and other conditions
  stanfordhealthcare.org

- Alzheimer's Foundation of America
  Caregiving support, education, memory screening
  www.alzfdn.org

- Alzheimer's Research & Prevention Foundation
  Research, training, prevention, memory screening
  www.alzheimersprevention.org

- Family Caregiver Alliance
  General information, caregiving resources, support groups
  www.caregiver.org

Other Caregiving Resources

- Alzheimer's & Dementia Weekly
  General information, guidance
  www.alzheimersweekly.com

- Your Alzheimer's Community
  Resources, information, guidance
  www.alzheimers.net

- National Caregivers Library
  General information, resources, checklists
  www.caregiverslibrary.org

- AgingCare
  Newsletters, forum, support
  www.agingcare.com

- American Association of Retired Persons, AARP
  General information, family caregiving
  www.aarp.org/caregiving
  www.aarp.org/home-family/caregiving

- SeniorsMatter
  Resources, information, guidance
  www.seniorsmatter.com

- HelpGuide
  General information, mental health, wellness, aging
  www.helpguide.org

Legal

- FindLaw
  Information, find an elder lawyer in your city
  www.findlaw.com/elder

- National Elder Law Foundation
  Information, directory of certified elder law attorneys
  nelf.org

Books

- The 36-Hour Day: a Family Guide to Caring for Persons with
  Alzheimer's Disease, Related Dementing Illnesses, and Memory
  Loss in Later Life
  Mace, Nancy L.
  Baltimore: Johns Hopkins University Press, 1981.

- What If It's Not Alzheimer's? A Caregiver's Guide to Dementia
  Radin, Lisa, and Gary Radin, Editors
  Prometheus Books, 2003.

- Gone From my Sight: the Dying Experience
  Karnes, Barbara
  Vancouver, WA: Barbara Karnes Books, 1986.

- Still Alice: a Novel
  Genova, Lisa
  New York: Pocket Books, 2010.

REFERENCES

Accurate Hearing, (n.d.), "Hearing Loss Associated with Increased Risk of Dementia," Accessed Nov 25, 2021, from https://accuratehearing.ca/hearing-loss-associated-with-increased-risk-of-dementia/

Alzheimer's Association, (n.d.), "Types of Dementia, Lewy Body Dementia," Accessed Nov 25, 2021, from https://www.alz.org/alzheimers-dementia/what-is-dementia/types-of-dementia/lewy-body-dementia

Alzheimer's Association, (n.d.), "Types of Dementia, Vascular Dementia," Accessed Nov 25, 2021, from https://www.alz.org/alzheimers-dementia/what-is-dementia/types-of-dementia/vascular-dementia

Alzheimer's Association, (n.d.), "Wandering", Accessed Nov 25, 2021 from https://www.alz.org/help-support/caregiving/stages-behaviors/wandering

Alzheimer's Society, (n.d.), "Non-drug Approaches to Changes in Mood and Behavior," Accessed Nov 25, 2021 from https://www.alzheimers.org.uk/about-dementia/treatments/drugs/non-drug-approaches-changes-mood-and-behaviour

Alzheimer's & Dementia Weekly, (n.d.), "Red Plates for Eating with Dementia," Accessed Nov 25, 2021, from http://www.alzheimersweekly.com/2014/08/red-plates-for-eating-with-dementia.html

Ancelin, M. L., G. De Roquefeuil, and K. Ritchie. "Anesthesia and postoperative cognitive dysfunction in the elderly: a review of clinical and epidemiological observations." *Revue D'epidemiologie et de Sante Publique* 48.5 (2000): 459-472.

Baker, John, et al. "The prevalence and clinical features of epileptic seizures in a memory clinic population." *Seizure* 71 (2019): 83-92.

Blundon, Elizabeth G., Romayne E. Gallagher, and Lawrence M. Ward. "Electrophysiological evidence of preserved hearing at the end of life." *Scientific reports* 10.1 (2020): 1-13.

Boger, Jennifer, Tammy Craig, and Alex Mihailidis. "Examining the impact of familiarity on faucet usability for older adults with dementia." *BMC geriatrics* 13.1 (2013): 1-12.

Byeon, Gihwan, et al. "Dual sensory impairment and cognitive impairment in the Korean Longitudinal Elderly Cohort." *Neurology* 96.18 (2021): e2284-e2295.

Chen, Jen-Hau, Kun-Pei Lin, and Yen-Ching Chen. "Risk factors for dementia." *Journal of the Formosan Medical Association* 108.10 (2009): 754-764.

Clarke, Diana E., et al. "Apathy in dementia: clinical and sociodemographic correlates." *The Journal of neuropsychiatry and clinical neurosciences* 20.3 (2008): 337-347.

Coburn, Mark, A. Fahlenkamp, and Norbert Zoremba. (Feb 2010), "Postoperative Cognitive Dysfunction: Incidence and Prophylaxis," ResearchGate, Accessed Nov 25, 2021 from https://www.researchgate.net/publication/41056915_Postoperative_cognitive_dysfunction_Incidence_and_prophylaxis

Cooper, Claudia, Amber Selwood, and Gill Livingston. "The prevalence of elder abuse and neglect: a systematic review." *Age and ageing* 37.2 (2008): 151-160.

Custodio, Nilton, et al. "Mixed dementia: A review of the evidence." *Dementia & neuropsychologia* 11 (2017): 364-370.

De Giorgi, Riccardo, and Hugh Series. "Treatment of inappropriate sexual behavior in dementia." *Current treatment options in neurology* 18.9 (2016): 1-15.

Dementia Organization; (n.d.), "Frontotemporal Dementia Facts," Accessed Nov 25, 2021, from https://www.dementia.org/frontotemporal-dementia-facts

Dennis, Jacqueline. "Changing our view of older people's continence care." *Nursing Times* 112.20 (2016): 12-14.

Desai, Roopal, et al. "Living alone and risk of dementia: A systematic review and meta-analysis." *Ageing Research Reviews* 62 (2020): 101122.

Donovan, Nancy J., et al. "Regional cortical thinning predicts worsening apathy and hallucinations across the Alzheimer disease spectrum." *The American Journal of Geriatric Psychiatry* 22.11 (2014): 1168-1179.

Drennan, Vari M., et al. "Conservative interventions for incontinence in people with dementia or cognitive impairment, living at home: a systematic review." *BMC Geriatrics* 12.1 (2012): 1-10.

Fader, Mandy, et al. "Continence products: research priorities to improve the lives of people with urinary and/or fecal leakage." *Neurourology and Urodynamics: Official Journal of the International Continence Society* 29.4 (2010): 640-644.

Fleming, Richard, Fiona Kelly, and Gillian Stillfried. "'I want to feel at home': establishing what aspects of environmental design are important to people with dementia nearing the end of life." *BMC Palliative Care* 14.1 (2015): 1-14.

Flinker, Adeen, et al. "Redefining the role of Broca's area in speech." *Proceedings of the National Academy of Sciences* 112.9 (2015): 2871-2875.

Franx, Bart AA, et al. "Weight loss in patients with dementia: considering the potential impact of pharmacotherapy." *Drugs & aging* 34.6 (2017): 425-436.

Furlanetto, Kate, and Katherine Emond. "'Will I come home incontinent?' A retrospective file review: Incidence of development of incontinence and correlation with length of stay in acute settings for people with dementia or cognitive impairment aged 65 years and over." *Collegian* 23.1 (2016): 79-86.

Gaugler, Joseph E., et al. "Consistency of dementia caregiver intervention classification: an evidence-based synthesis." *International Psychogeriatrics* 29.1 (2017): 19-30.

Genova, Lisa. *Still Alice: a Novel.* New York: Pocket Books, 2010.

Gitlin, Laura N., Helen C. Kales, and Constantine G. Lyketsos. "Managing behavioral symptoms in dementia using nonpharmacologic approaches: an overview." *JAMA: the journal of the American Medical Association* 308.19 (2012): 2020.

Hulse, Gary K., et al. "Dementia associated with alcohol and other drug use." *International Psychogeriatrics* 17.s1 (2005): S109-S127.

Hwang, Jen-Ping, et al. "Hoarding behavior in dementia: A preliminary report." *The American Journal of Geriatric Psychiatry* 6.4 (1998): 285-289.

Hwang, Phillip H. "Double Trouble: Impact of Hearing, Vision Loss on Dementia Risk." *The Hearing Journal* 73.10 (2020): 8-9.

Johannesen, Mark, and Dina LoGiudice. "Elder abuse: A systematic review of risk factors in community-dwelling elders." *Age and ageing* 42.3 (2013): 292-298.

Joling, Karlijn J., et al. "Factors of resilience in informal caregivers of people with dementia from integrative international data analysis." *Dementia and Geriatric Cognitive Disorders* 42.3-4 (2016): 198-214.

Kales, Helen C., et al. "Management of neuropsychiatric symptoms of dementia in clinical settings: recommendations from a multidisciplinary expert panel." *Journal of the American Geriatrics Society* 62.4 (2014): 762-769.

Kang, Hyo Shin, et al. "Comparison of neuropsychological profiles in patients with Alzheimer's disease and mixed dementia." *Journal of the neurological sciences* 369 (2016): 134-138.

Karnes, Barbara. *Gone From my Sight: the Dying Experience.* Vancouver, WA: Barbara Karnes Books, 1986.

Kojima, Gotaro, et al. "Frailty as a predictor of Alzheimer disease, vascular dementia, and all dementia among community-dwelling older people: a systematic review and meta-analysis." *Journal of the American Medical Directors Association* 17.10 (2016): 881-888.

Lai, Michelle. (Jan 28, 2014), "How to Manage Teeth Grinding (Bruxism) in Dementia," slideshare, Accessed Nov 25, 2021) from https://www.slideshare.net/MichelleLai1/bruxism-in-dementia-lai-adi-poster-2013

Livingston, Gill, et al. "Dementia prevention, intervention, and care: 2020 report of the Lancet Commission." *The Lancet* 396.10248 (2020): 413-446.

Logsdon, Rebecca G., Susan M. McCurry, and Linda Teri. "Evidence-based interventions to improve quality of life for individuals with dementia." *Alzheimer's care today* 8.4 (2007): 309.

Louis, Elan D., and Stephan A. Mayer. *Merritt's Neurology.* Lippincott Williams & Wilkins, 2021.

Mace, Nancy L. "The 36-Hour Day: a Family Guide to Caring for Persons with Alzheimer's Disease, Related Dementing Illnesses, and Memory Loss in Later Life." Baltimore: Johns Hopkins University Press, 1981.

Macpherson, Helen, et al. "The Influence of the Mediterranean Diet on Cognitive Health." *The Mediterranean Diet* (2015): 81-89.

Majlesi, Ali Reza, and Anna Ekström. "Baking together—the coordination of actions in activities involving people with dementia." *Journal of Aging Studies* 38 (2016): 37-46.

Mathew, Thomas, Shruthi Venkatesh, and Meghana Srinivas. "The approach and management of bruxism in Alzheimer's disease: An under-recognized habit that concerns caregivers (innovative practice)." *Dementia* 19.2 (2020): 461-463.

Müller-Spahn, Franz. "Behavioral disturbances in dementia." *Dialogues in clinical neuroscience* (2022).

National Institute on Aging, (n.d.), "How Is Alzheimer's Disease Treated?," Accessed Jun 28, 2022, from https://www.nia.nih.gov/ health/how-alzheimers-disease-treated

National Institute on Aging, (n.d.), "What Do We Know About Diet and Prevention of Alzheimer's Disease?" Accessed Jun 28, 2022, from https://www.nia.nih.gov/health/what-do-we-know-about-diet-and-prevention-alzheimers-disease

O'neill, Desmond, et al. "Dementia and driving." *Journal of the Royal Society of Medicine* 85.4 (1992): 199.

Ostaszkiewicz, Joan, Tracey Chestney, and Brenda Roe. "Habit retraining for the management of urinary incontinence in adults." *Cochrane Database of Systematic Reviews* 2 (2004).

Peterson, Kendra, et al. "In the Information Age, do dementia caregivers get the information they need? Semi-structured interviews to determine informal caregivers' education needs, barriers, and preferences." *BMC geriatrics* 16.1 (2016): 1-13.

Politzer, Thomas. (Nov 2008) "Vision Is Our Dominant Sense", brainline, Accessed Nov 25, 2021 from https://www.brainline.org/article/vision-our-dominant-sense

Qiu, Chengxuan, Miia Kivipelto, and Eva Von Strauss. "Epidemiology of Alzheimer's disease: occurrence, determinants, and strategies toward intervention." *Dialogues in clinical neuroscience* (2022).

Radin, Lisa, and Gary Radin, Editors. *What If It's Not Alzheimer's? A Caregiver's Guide to Dementia.* Prometheus Books, 2003.

Rochester Review. (Mar-April 2012), "The Mind's Eye" Rochester Review, Vol 74 No 4, accessed Nov 20, 2021, from https://www.rochester.edu/pr/Review/V74N4/0402_brainscience.html

Sampson, Elizabeth L., Bridget Candy, and Louise Jones. "Enteral tube feeding for older people with advanced dementia." *Cochrane database of systematic reviews* 2 (2009).

Schulz, Richard, and Scott R. Beach. "Caregiving as a risk factor for mortality: the Caregiver Health Effects Study." *JAMA* 282.23 (1999): 2215-2219.

Stanford Health Care, (n.d.), "Dementia Risk Factors," Accessed Nov 25, 2021, from https://stanfordhealthcare.org/medical-conditions/brain-and-nerves/dementia/risk-factors.html

Tanaka, Kumiko, et al. "Factors related to the urination methods of elderly people with incontinence who require at-home nursing care." *Nihon Ronen Igakkai zasshi. Japanese Journal of Geriatrics* 53.2 (2016): 133-142.

The Recovery Village (Apr 2021) "Dementia and Substance Abuse," Accessed Nov 2021 from https://www.therecoveryvillage.com/mental-health/dementia/substance-abuse/

Turró-Garriga, Oriol, et al. "Consequences of anosognosia on the cost of caregivers' care in Alzheimer's disease." *Journal of Alzheimer's Disease* 54.4 (2016): 1551-1560.

University College London (July 30, 2020), "Four in Ten Dementia Cases Could Be Prevented or Delayed," UCL News, Accessed Nov 20, 2021, from https://www.ucl.ac.uk/news/2020/jul/four-10-dementia-cases-could-be-prevented-or-delayed

U.S. Access Board, (n.d.), "Guide to the ADA Accessibility Standards, Chapter 4: Ramps and Curb Ramps" Accessed Jun 27, 2022, from https://www.access-board.gov/ada/guides/chapter-4-ramps-and-curb-ramps/

Wanko Keutchafo, Esther L., Jane Kerr, and Mary Ann Jarvis. "Evidence of nonverbal communication between nurses and older adults: a scoping review." *BMC nursing* 19.1 (2020): 1-13.

Wetzels, R. B., et al. "Prescribing pattern of psychotropic drugs in nursing home residents with dementia." *International psychogeriatrics* 23.8 (2011): 1249-1259.

Yoon, Kyung Hee, et al. "The moderating effect of religiosity on caregiving burden and depressive symptoms in caregivers of patients with dementia." *Aging & Mental Health* 22.1 (2018): 141-147.

Zwerling, Jessica L., Jason A. Cohen, and Joe Verghese. "Dementia and caregiver stress." *Neurodegenerative disease management* 6.2 (2016): 69-72.

INDEX

ACKNOWLEDGEMENT

This book is an outgrowth of my work with the Dardashna Project, an educational and advocacy project for dementia caregivers in Persian. This book, and indeed the Dardashna Project as a whole, has benefited greatly from the support and encouragement of many individuals from across the dementia landscape, whose contributions have enriched the project in immeasurable ways.

I especially wish to thank H. A. Ebrahimi, Professor of Neurology at Kerman Medical Sciences University (KMU), K. Bahaadini, Assistant Professor of Medical Informatics at KMU, Sh. Mazhari, Assistant Professor of Psychiatry at KMU, and M. Nowroozian, Professor of Neurology at Tehran Medical Sciences University, for their unfailing support throughout the project. I would like to thank especially K. Shafiee, Assistant Professor of Neurology at KMU, for his painstaking review of evolving manuscripts for medical accuracy, J. Khoshamooz and M. Samadani for their tireless efforts in editing and organizing the final manuscript, E. F. DeLiso and S. D. Johnson for copy editing, and E. Azarnoosh and R. Kear for bringing the book to life with their artistry.

This book owes its soul to the countless caregivers who shared their struggles and their wisdom so that others can benefit from their experiences. Caring for a loved one with dementia is a labor of love and silent sacrifice. It is their love and sacrifice that breathes through the pages of this book.

Finally, a word of thanks to my wife: the love of my life and my companion, confidant, and trusted adviser throughout our shared journey. None of this would have been possible without her. Indeed, it was her illness and our joint struggle with dementia as patient and caregiver that was the spark for much that followed since, including this book.

About the Author

Mehdi Samadani spent his career in the tech industry. He has held positions from engineering to management and corporate governance, including a stint as lecturer at IBM's International Education Center in La Hulpe, Belgium. He is the founder of the Dardashna Project (literally, "One who knows pain"), an educational and advocacy project for dementia caregivers in Persian. He has coauthored three previous books on dementia caregiving in Farsi, which have been peer reviewed by faculty at the departments of neurology and psychiatry of Kerman Medical Sciences University, and published under the auspices of that institution. He has written more than 150 articles covering all aspects of dementia caregiving, which are available for free at the Dardashna Project website. He manages the Dardashna caregiving forum and support groups. He has been a caregiver for seventeen years.

Printed in Great Britain
by Amazon

58208006R00235